HELLO!
MY REAL NAME IS...

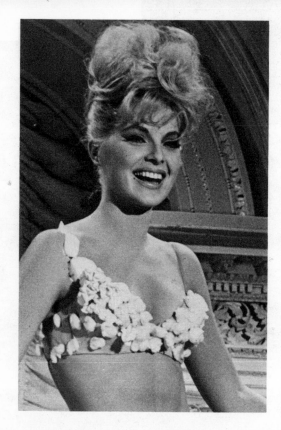

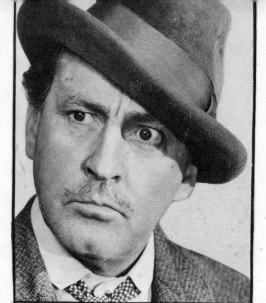

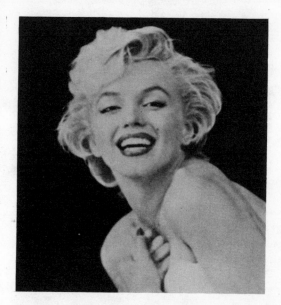

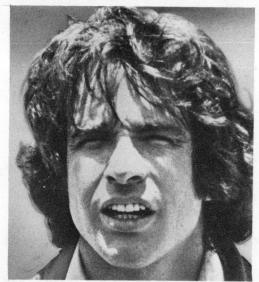

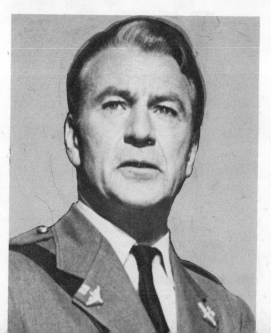

BOOKS BY THE SAME AUTHOR

The Chutspah Book
Some of My Best Friends Are People
Pros and Cons
The Complete Pun Book
Hello! My Real Name Is. . . .

HELLO!
MY REAL NAME IS...

ART. MOGER

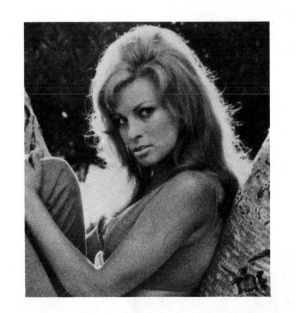

CITADEL PRESS   Seacaucus, N.J.

First edition
Copyright © 1983 by Art. Moger
All rights reserved
Published by Citadel Press
A division of Lyle Stuart Inc.
120 Enterprise Ave., Secaucus, N.J. 07094
In Canada: Musson Book Company
A division of General Publishing Co. Limited
Don Mills, Ontario
Manufactured in the United States of America
Designed by Christopher Simon
ISBN 0-8065-0802-7

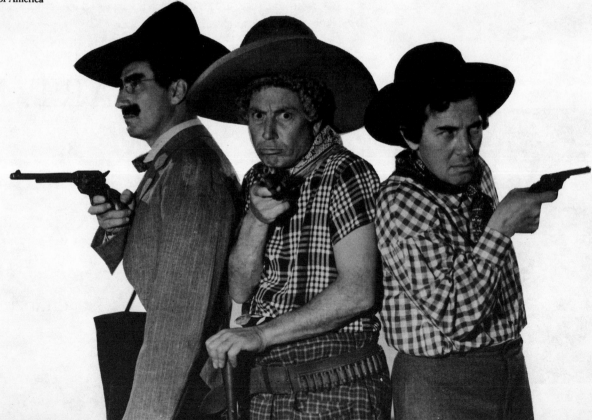

Dedicated to
MY WIFE, DORA—
(aka) "Dodo"
who, by any other name,
would be *"Dear"*

CONTENTS

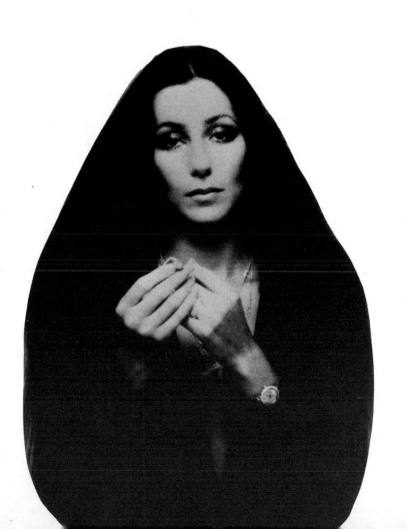

Sticks and stones
May break my bones,
But names
Will never hurt me

       —CHILDREN'S DOGGEREL

8

"A man, if acting honestly, may assume any name he desires and by which he wishes to be known in the community in which he lives or in the trade circles in which he does business. The law does not require a man to retain and to perpetuate the surname of his ancestors. The common law recognizes his freedom of choice to assume a name which he deems more appropriate and advantageous to him than his family name in his present circumstances, if the change is not motivated by fraudulent intent."

"It is well settled that at common law a person may change his name at will, without resort to legal proceedings, by merely adopting another name, provided that this is done for an honest purpose. (Massachusetts has a statute which prescribes the method by which a name can be changed with legal effect.) But it does not follow that one may not assume or use another name without resort to the statute if such use is for an honest purpose. In numerous cases decided after the passage of the statute it has been recognized that without compliance with it one may use another name for transacting business, making contracts, instituting or defending law suits, and acquiring and transferring title to property, where such use is not tainted by fraud."

The above quotation is from the Supreme Judicial Court of Massachusetts case of:

Frank Buyarsky & others, petitioners recorded in Volume 322 Mass. reports at page 336. The opinion was written by Judge James J. Ronan on February 2, 1948. (Frank Buyarsky became Frank Byers.)

The above quotation is from a decision of the Supreme Judicial Court of Massachusetts in the case of *Israel Merolevitz & others, petitioners*, and written by Judge John Varnum Spalding in 320 of the Massachusetts reports at page 450 (decided November 29, 1946).

(Israel Merolevitz became Irving Merrill).

Names are not made in Heaven. Witness this!

God is alive and well and living in Fresno, California.

Terrill Clark Williams, a writer and one-time broadcaster, became "God" in the eyes of the law, recently, when Superior Court Judge Charles Hamlin signed the official decrees of name change.

Williams didn't find it easy to become "God." He couldn't get a lawyer to handle the court petition because they said no judge would sign it. He then had to give up his job because his superiors were uncomfortable with his idea.

"I'm not breaking the Second Commandment by taking the Lord's name in vain," said Williams—er—*God*, that is.

"I'm praising the Lord by taking his name."

The only problem *God* has is that as Terrill Clark Williams, people would say: "God bless you," when he sneezed.

What do they say now, when *God* sneezes?

LIVING IT UP

GEORGE BURNS

Let me tell you a little about myself. I never played a good theater until I met Gracie. Before that I was a small-time vaudeville actor until I was twenty-seven years old. You should have seen some of the broken-down theaters I played. I played one theater that was so bad "Madame Burkhardt and Her Cockatoos" were the headliners. I was just unbelievably bad, but who cared. I wanted to be in show business and I was. I had to change my name every week. I could never get a job with the same name twice. I was Jack Harris of Harris & Kelly. I was Phil Baxter of Baxter & Bates. I was Davis of Delight and Davis—my name was Sammy Davis. Don't look so shocked. I was Jewish before he was, too. I used so many different names I got to the point where I didn't know who I was.

I remember one of the first acts I ever did was a singing, dancing and rollerskating act—Brown and Williams. Sid Brown and Harry Williams. . . . I don't remember whether I was Brown or Williams, but we got into a fight and split up the act. We both got different partners, and again we all did the same act. Now we had Brown and Williams, Williams and Brown, Brown and Brown and Williams and Williams, the Brown Brothers, and the Williams Boys. By the time we got through, every Jewish person on the East Side was either named Brown or Williams. There was one kid, Hymie Goldberg, he moved. He said he was afraid to live in a gentile neighborhood.

Then I did a ballroom dancing act called Pedro Lopez and Conchita. My name was Pedro Lopez. Conchita's real name was Lila Berkowitz, but I used to smoke those little Conchita cigars, so I named her after the cigar. . . . We were booked into the Farley Theater in Brooklyn, and to give you an idea of how bad we were, the music for our opening number was "La Czarina," which is a Russian mazurka. We thought it was a Spanish dance, so we wore Spanish outfits. I wore a little black bolero coat with a green sash around my waist, and I parted my hair in the middle and plastered it down with Vaseline. I wanted to look like Ramon Navarro. . . .

Conchita had a red Spanish shawl with gold fringe around it, which she'd fasten under one arm, leaving one shoulder bare. And she wore one of those big, heavy Spanish combs in her hair. It used to press on a nerve in her head and drove her crazy—they finally had to take her away. . . . She wore an evening dress under the shawl, and for our second number she'd pull the shawl off and put her arm in the sleeve of her dress. Then she'd pick up a fan, and she was ready. I'd pull off my sash, put on a top hat, grab my cane, and we were ready to do our next number, which was a Cakewalk.

At this one particular performance that comb was pressing on Conchita's nerve, and she didn't know what she was doing. She picked up her fan okay, but when she took off the shawl she forgot to put her arm in her sleeve. Well, when we started the Cakewalk, which is a very bouncy number, with her arm out of her sleeve, one of her things kept flapping up against her chest. I thought it was the audience applauding, so I kept taking bows.

Our closing number was a Turkey Trot with a whirlwind finish. For this Conchita had changed into a white evening gown with just two thin straps. Now, Conchita came from the lower East Side, and in those days a lot of Jewish girls never shaved under their arms, so she had all this hair hanging down. When we started to pivot, with that comb pressing on her nerve and me stepping on her hair, poor Conchita was sorry she ever got into show business. And for our finish she'd put her arms around my neck and I'd spin her around in the air. It looked like I was swinging two rabbis. Anyway, before the week was over they took Conchita away, and I changed my name again.

INTRODUCTION, WHAT'S IN A NAME?

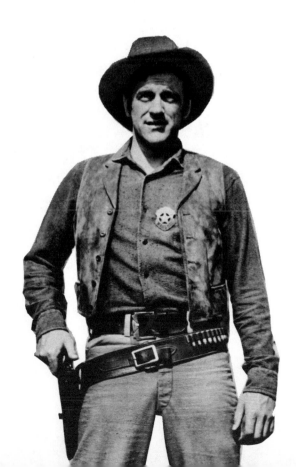

One afternoon, a young actor named Louis Morelli walked into an office in Hollywood. When he walked out, his name was *Trax Colton*. No one had ever heard of him before, and no one has heard of him since. But he has at least taken a minor place in an ancient rite of Hollywood. Moreover, Morelli was restyled by one of the wizard name-changers practicing the craft—Agent Henry Willson, the man who christened the *reel* names of Rhonda Fleming, Rory Calhoun, Tab Hunter, Guy Madison and—his great mind wandering from the New Jersey Palisades to the Straits of Gibraltar—Rock Hudson.

In show business the *reel* name supplants the *real* name before the actor's teeth are capped. Hundreds of literary types like Willson have, over the years, flung into the air a confetti storm of phony names that have settled meaningfully onto American Culture. Names have had to be shortened (there is a group called the *readily understandable*). Some lacked euphony. Others sounded too ethnic. So there came to be such great show business celebrities as: Kirk Douglas, Cyd Charisse, Judy Garland, Mickey Rooney, Ann Miller, Jane Wyman, Judy Holliday, Red Buttons, John Wayne, Danny Kaye, Jack Benny, Fred Allen, Jerry Lewis, Dean Martin, Bo Derek, William Holden, Doris Day, Cary Grant, Danny Thomas, Ann Sothern, Susan Hayward and hundreds of others. *None of them became famous using his or her real names!*

Did you know that Lawrence Welk is his *real* name?

There are hundreds of unusual photographs in this unusual book of people who were well-known by their *reel* names. But will you recognize the names given to them at birth? You'll be genuinely surprised at your lack of accuracy. Don't feel discouraged. Many will learn for the first time that their favorite movie stars were born with a name different from what they are known by.

There are three names below each photograph. Only *one* is correct. If you are stumped, the correct answers are in the back of the book. *No cheating, please!* You'll also learn plenty of trivia which will rarely come up in conversation, unless you start it first.

As my late friend, cartoonist Al Capp, said: "It's amusin' but confusin'!" *Good luck!*

January 1983   THE AUTHOR
Boston, Massachusetts

ACKNOWLEDGMENTS

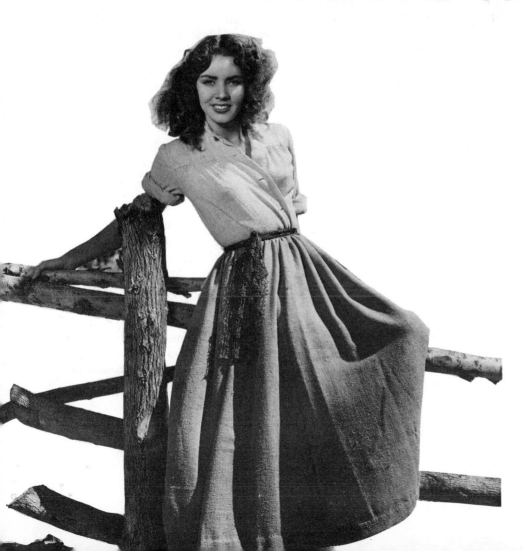

15

Credit—Where Credit Is Due

My sincerest thanks to the scores of friends who have contributed their unselfish efforts on behalf of this gigantic research project, supplying me with photographs, data, biographies, *real/reel* names and other information appearing herein. I have tried to include all who have made this book possible. If I've omitted any names it's because my memory isn't what it used to be. Besides, this book would have been much thinner without everyone's help.

Thank you!

You know who you are, which is more than the personalities shown in the ensuing pages can say for themselves.

Names are not always what they seem to be. The common Welch name "Bzjxxllwcp" is pronounced "Jackson." (Are you listenin', Reggie?) The first Rotarian was the first man to call John the Baptist *Jack!*

Who will ever forget the endearing lines uttered by Romeo to his beloved Juliet, *"What's in a name? That which we call a rose by any other name would smell as sweet."* Juliet might have replied, facetiously, *"There is everything in a name. A rose by any other name would smell as sweet but would not cost half as much during the winter months."*

There seems to be a marked rivalry among people to get their names listed first in their respective telephone directories. For example, the first name in the Boston and New York directories is the letter "A." Probably the longest and oddest name appeared in the Manhattan telephone book. It was "Zzherobrouskievskieskieea." His friends call him just plain "Mr. Z."

I am deeply indebted to THE Paul Sullivan, talented journalist/columnist of THE PAGE, in the *Boston Herald/American*; Robert A. Parsons, Boston, Mass.; Hon. A. Alan Friedberg, president, Sack Theaters, Boston, Mass.; Susan Fraine, PR director, Sack Theaters, Boston, Mass.; Sherry Natkow, Sack Theaters, Boston, Mass.; Stanley H. Moger, president, SFM Holiday Network, New York; Maria "Mattie" Matlaga, of Carteret, N.J.; Harry D. Trigg, pioneer motion picture/TV expert and Program Manager, WGN-TV, Chicago, Ill.; Henry Luhrman Associates, New York; Ruth Webb, Ruth Webb Enterprises, Los Angeles, Calif.; *Living It Up* by George Burns, reprinted by permission of G. P. Putnam's Sons from LIVING IT UP by George Burns, copyright © 1976 by George Burns; Sam and Corinne Dame, Lordly & Dame, Inc., Boston, Mass.; Hon. Nathan Moger, prominent Boston attorney, for his legal expertise; *Motion Picture Almanac*; Bill Devine and Ellen Yoerger, Hub Mail, Inc., Boston, Mass.; Val Almendarez, Academy of Motion Picture Arts and Sciences, Beverly Hills, Calif.; artist Bernie Weinstock, Boston, Mass.; Fred MacNeill, Concord, Mass.; Doug Dame, Dame Associates, Boston, Mass.; W. S. Bernheimer II, for yours truly's photo on back cover; Rosalind Bernheimer, Waban, Mass.; Harriet M. Watson, Portland, Oregon; Hank Grant, *The Hollywood Reporter*, Hollywood, Calif.; Boston Public Library, Humanities Dept.; Boston, Mass.; and last, but not least, publisher Allan J. Wilson of Citadel Press, Secaucus, N.J., who, like his namesake, agent Henry Willson (but with one "l"), is a namechanger, par excellence. Allan forsook my title, *Name Dropper*, in favor of his *"Hello! My Real Name Is . . ."* (*I like it, better!*) The format and layout is Wilson's, too. (*I like that, too!*)

All of this material has been culled from many reliable sources. It is as accurate as humanly possible. If there are any errors, the author and publisher express their regrets and offer their apologies. Maybe the corrections (if there are many) will appear in a sequel titled: *"Hello! My real Real Name Was . . ."*

Enough of this folderol. Match the photographs to their *real* names. You say it's easy? *Try it!* It's more fun than watching your neighbors' kids' camp pictures—and just as exhausting.

COL. ART. MOGER

1. SUPERSTARS

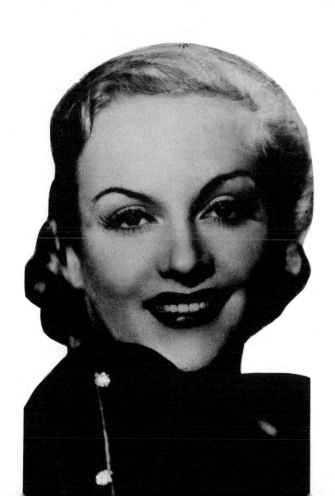

First name the celebrity, then guess his or her real name from the list that follows. Answers will be found in the back of the book.

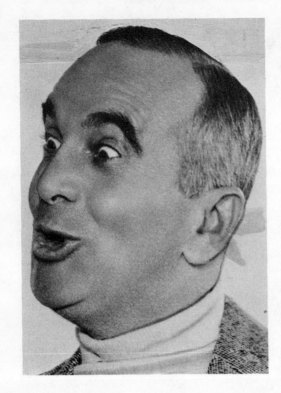

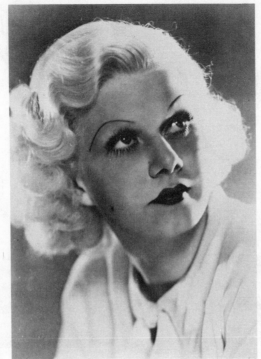

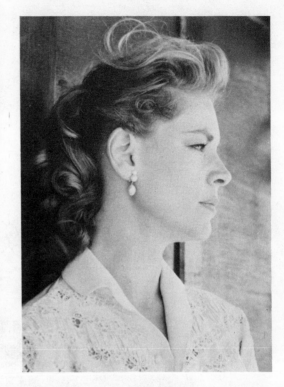

1

Some called him "the greatest entertainer in the world." He starred in *The Jazz Singer*, one of the screen's earliest talking motion pictures. He was a big stage and TV star, too.

1. *Alfred Sherman.*   2. *Asa Yoelson.*
3. *Allan Jolie.*

2

This blond bombshell became a sex symbol to millions during the early thirties. She was nicknamed "The Platinum Blonde."

1. *Blanche Urban.*   2. *Harlean Carpenter.*
3. *Jean Glowhardt.*

3

She is a sultry American actress equally at home on the stage or screen. She was married to Humphrey Bogart and Jason Robards.

1. *Lauren Feldman.*   2. *Bonnie Brooks.*
3. *Betty Joan Perske.*

18

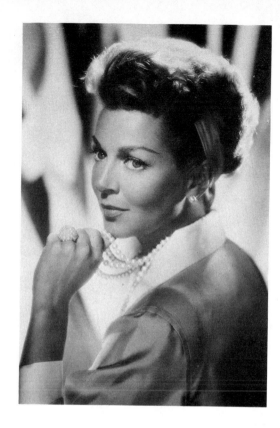

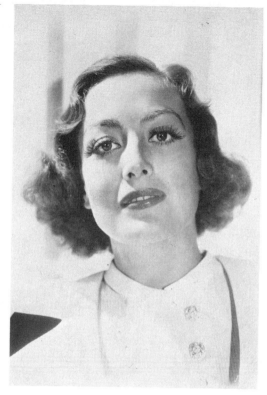

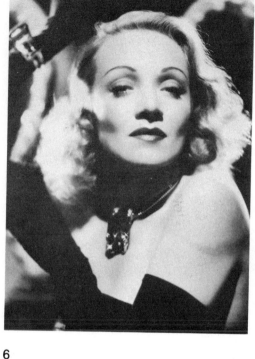

4

Probably one of the greatest sex symbols of her generation. She began as "the girl next door" type but became increasingly sophisticated.

1. *Robin Lyn Moger.*   2. *Barbara B. Parsons.*
3. *Julia Turner.*

5

She was known for a time as "Billie Cassin." She won an Academy Award for her role in *Mildred Pierce.*

1. *Niki Friedberg.*   2. *Lucille LeSueur.*
3. *Beth Blankstein.*

6

This glamorous singer-actress from Germany became a legend of sophistication on the American screen. She was also a fine singer, especially in *Blue Angel.* She was excellent in *Witness for the Prosecution.*

1. *Marlene Deutsch.*   2. *Jo Somers.*
3. *Maria Magdalena von Losch.*

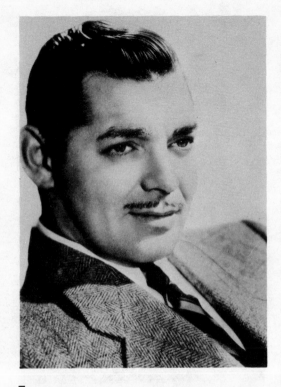

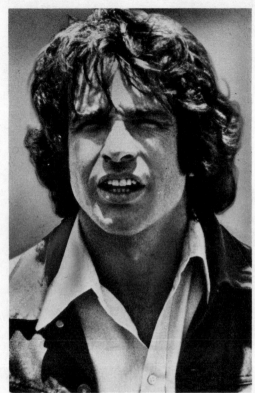

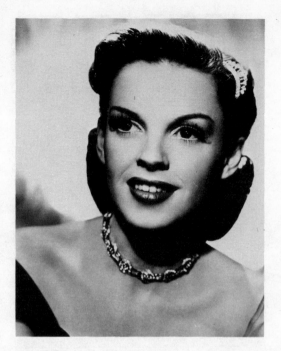

7

Probably the best-liked leading man in motion pictures, whose macho image, on the screen, made him the idol of millions. He was best known for his role as "Rhett Butler" in *Gone With the Wind*. He was affectionately known as "The King."

1. *Paul J. Carnese.*   2. *William C. Gable.*
3. *Gable Clarkson.*

8

This handsome leading man has captivated the hearts of millions of admirers. He produced as well as acted in *Shampoo*, and won an Oscar for his direction of *Reds*.

1. *Walter Beeson.*   2. *Barron Warren.*
3. *Warren Beaty.*

9

The one and only, she was given her screen name by George Jessel, who thought her real name was too common for moviegoers. She was on stage from the time she was five years old and radiated the soul of show business. She won a Special Oscar "for her outstanding performances as a juvenile," and captivated millions with her rendition of "Over the Rainbow."

1. *Faith Thomas.*   2. *Rosemary Alexander.*
3. *Frances Gumm.*

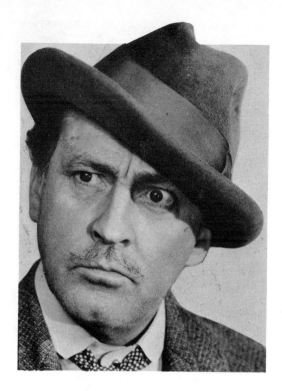

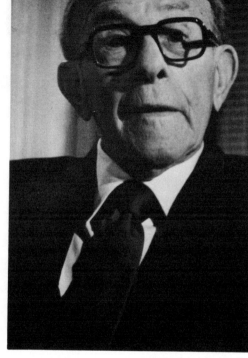

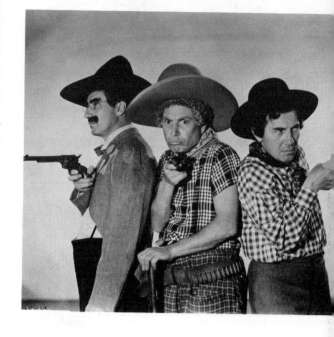

10

A great American character actor, and a celebrated stage and screen personality. He was known as "the great profile," and was as striking off as well as on stage or screen.

1. *John Blythe.* 2. *Gerald Williams.*
3. *Christopher Cross.*

This American vaudeville comedian married Gracie Allen and spent many successful years on radio and TV. An octogenarian, he still makes films, records songs, plays nightclubs, and appears on TV. He won an Oscar for his role in *The Sunshine Boys.*

1. *Nathan Birnbaum.* 2. *Marc Goldstein.*
3. *George Brown.*

12

Without a doubt the zaniest trio to appear on the stage or screen. Their films are among the funniest ever produced.

Groucho: 1. *Arthur.* 2. *Julius.* 3. *Stanley.*
Harpo: 1. *Adolph.* 2. *Peter.* 3. *Wally.*
Chico: 1. *Andy.* 2. *Eric.* 3. *Leonard.*

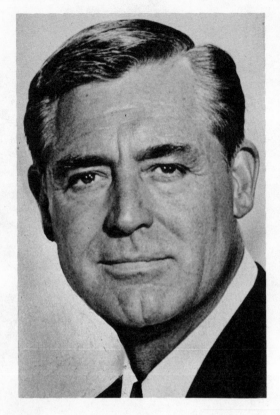

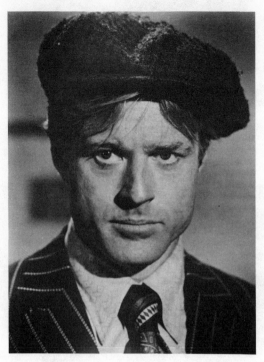

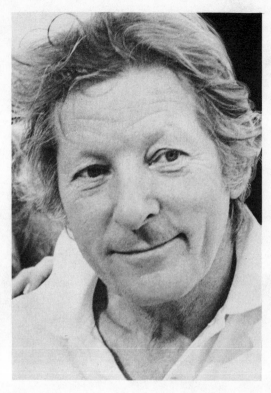

13

This debonair British-born leading man has a personality and accent all his own and has been the heartthrob of millions of moviegoers everywhere.

1. *Archibald Leach.* 2. *W. S. Bernheimer II.*
3. *Barney Frank.*

14

One of America's greatest leading men, who began as the leading man in the stage presentation of *Barefoot in the Park* and rose rapidly to stardom.

1. *Charles R. Redford, Jr.*
2. *Redford Charles II.*
3. *Bob King.*

15

One ot the most talented comedians of the musical comedy stage as well as films. He appears on TV and is a great champion of UNICEF.

1. *David Daniel Kaminsky.*
2. *Daniel Brotman.*
3. *Daniel Taylor.*

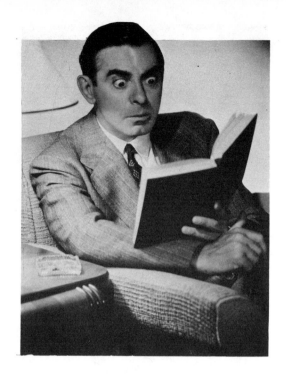 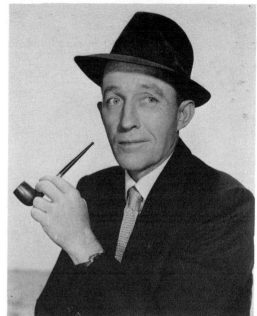 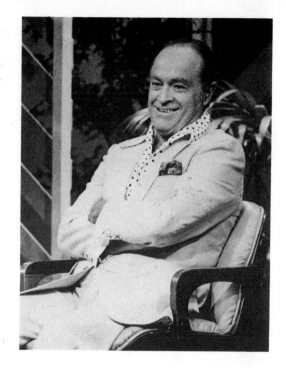

16

They called him "Banjo Eyes" on account of his rolling orbs. He was a great comedian of stage, vaudeville, screen, and radio/TV. He danced and sang as well.

1. *Ralph Dondero.*
2. *Edward Israel Iskowitz.*
3. *Israel Strier.*

17

He was a star crooner and a former band singer. Later he became a comedian and a romantic lead in films, winning an Oscar in *Going My Way*. He teamed with Bob Hope for a series of "Road" films which were very successful.

1. *Frank Hayes.*   2. *Roger Demaris.*
3. *Harry Lillis Crosby.*

18

One of the world's richest men, this amiable comedian has entertained troops with his inimitable shows, going into the most dangerous places with his contingents of entertainers. He is a star of films, stage, radio, and TV.

1. *Dick Baldwin.*   2. *Irwin Bogart.*
3. *Leslie Townes Hope.*

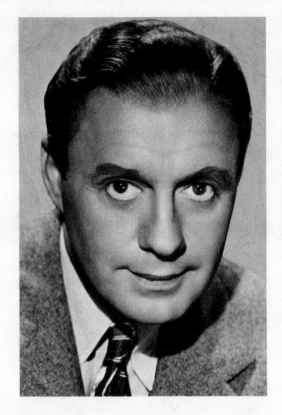

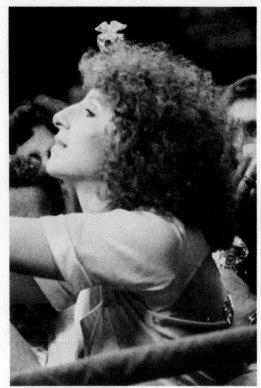

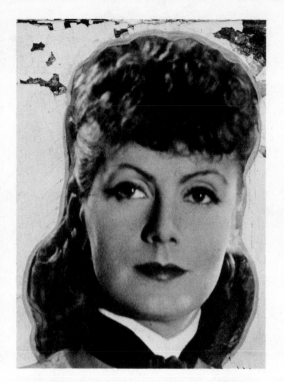

19

One of America's most beloved stars of stage, screen, radio, and TV. His mannerisms, such as just saying "Well!" could bring his audience to screaming laughter.

1. *Benjamin Kubelsky.*   2. *Jacob Benjamin.*
3. *Jack Benchick.*

20

One of the world's most successful songstresses and an Oscar winner for her film *Funny Girl*. A great comedienne and actress.

1. *Barbara Joan Streisand.*
2. *Susan Kate Moger.*
3. *Barbara Kempner.*

21

This glamorous Swedish actress was taken to Hollywood and became a goddess of the screen. She won a Special Academy Award for her unforgettable performances in such classics as *Camille*.

1. *Greta Louisa Gustafson.*
2. *Mary Lou Montanus.*
3. *Carol Lee Veitch.*

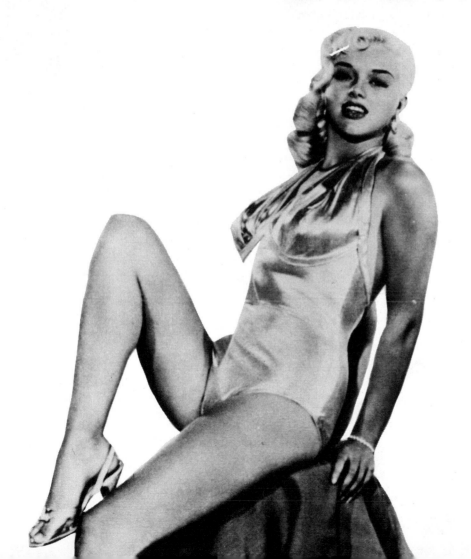

2. SEX SYMBOLS

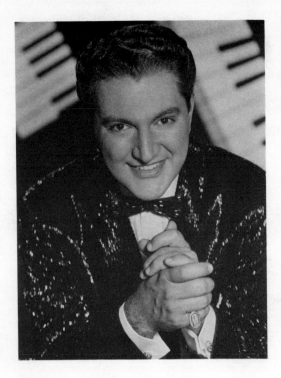

23

He's an American dancing star whose inimitable finesse and great sense of humor delighted millions for more than three decades. He and his dancing partner, Ginger Rogers, seemed to have a magic of their own.

1. *Robert Maxwell.*   2. *Frederick Austerlitz.*
3. *Fred Adair.*

24

She was a former band singer who had a brief stage career before going to Hollywood and achieving stardom with Fred Astaire. She won an Oscar for her role in *Kitty Foyle.*

1. *Virginia McMath.*   2. *Sue Carol Ladd.*
3. *Helen Gurley Brown.*

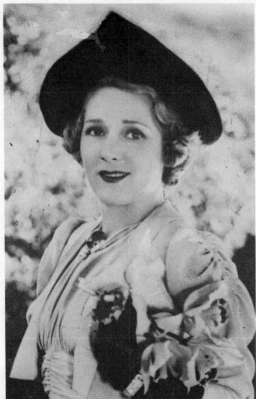

22

"Mr. Showbiz" himself, he is well known for his elaborate costumes, candelabra on the piano, and masterful piano technique. He is the darling of fashionable nightclubs in Las Vegas and has made a few films.

1. *Herman Liberace.*
2. *Wladziu Valentino Liberace.*
3. *Liberace Paderewski.*

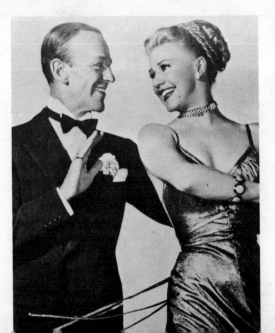

25

One of America's most beloved actresses of the silent screen. She was known as "America's Sweetheart."

1. *Anita MacNeill.*   2. *Gladys Smith.*
3. *Paula Henderson.*

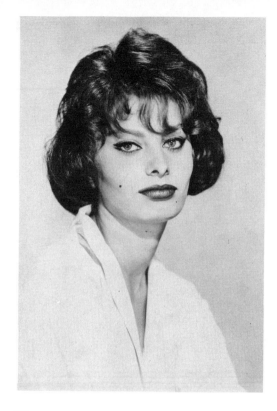

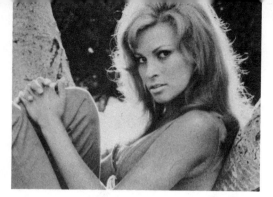

27

A great sex symbol and a dynamic and curvaceous actress who captivated audiences all over the world.

1. *Raquel Tejada.*   2. *Nancy Beth Goldstein.*
3. *Wendy Benerofe.*

28

This voluptuous Italian leading lady starred in innumerable spectacular films produced for the international market.

1. *Linda Bogart.*   2. *Sandi Maunello.*
                       3. *Virna Pieralisi.*

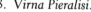

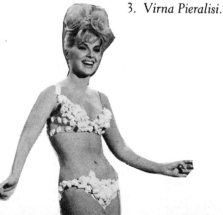

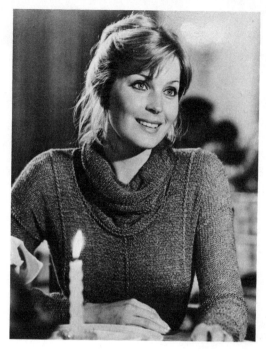

26

One of the great superstars of the screen, this beautiful Italian actress won an Oscar for *Two Women*.

1. *Sophia Lorenzo.*
2. *Sophia Scicoloni.*
3. *Sophie Stein.*

29

The film "*10*" made her name a household word. This beautiful actress is also a producer and has been acclaimed as one of the most beautiful women in the world.

1. *Mary Cathleen Collins.*
2. *Deborah Ann Bernheimer.*
3. *Harriet M. Watson.*

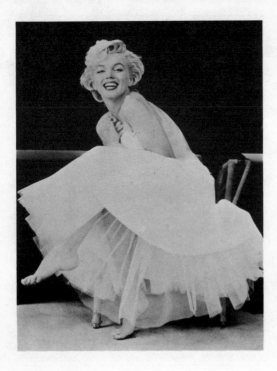

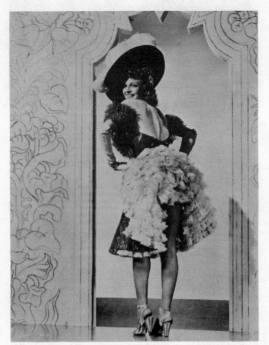

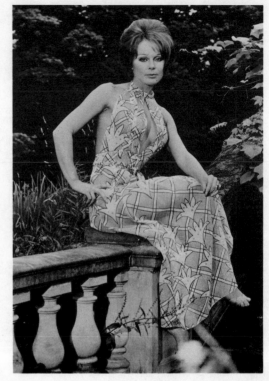

30

She was one of America's greatest sex symbols and the envy of millions until her demise. She rose from the ranks of models to become one of the world's greatest film superstars.

1. *Judy Brandman.* 2. *Norma Jean Baker.*
3. *Sarah Berwick.*

31

She was the darling of millions of GIs during World War II. This beautiful American leading lady was a brilliant dancer who often played tempestuous roles. She was on the stage from the age of six.

1. *Agatha Dorfman.*
2. *Margarita Carmen Cansino.*
3. *Doreen McInerney.*

32

This beautiful German actress has become an international star and appears frequently in Hollywood films and on TV. She is married to author-journalist Joe Hyams.

1. *Elke Schletz.* 2. *Paula Freedman.*
3. *Jody Davis.*

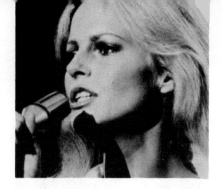

33

This beautiful blonde made her niche in *Charley's Angels* on TV. She is a talented singer and appears in nightclubs and on TV specials and records.

1. *Mary Sally Mergenthaler.*
2. *Cheryl Stoppelmoor.* 3. *Jane Tatarynowicz.*

34

This beautiful sex symbol was born in Mexico. At one time she was married to Tyrone Power, and is a cousin to screen actress Katy Jurado.

1. *Blanca Rosa Welter.* 2. *Shelly Schwab.*
3. *Cynthia Fischer.*

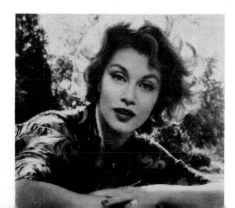

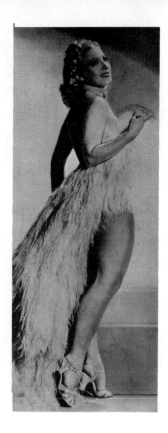

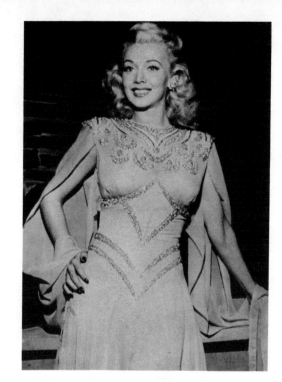

35

She was famous as the originator of the "Fan Dance" and made a few Hollywood films.

1. *Helen Gould Beck.*
2. *Debbie Spitaletta.*
3. *Sally Randall.*

36

She was a buxom, sultry American actress and leading lady during the forties.

1. *Frances Ridste.* 2. *Sue Weinstein.*
3. *Carol Landers.*

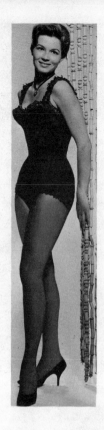

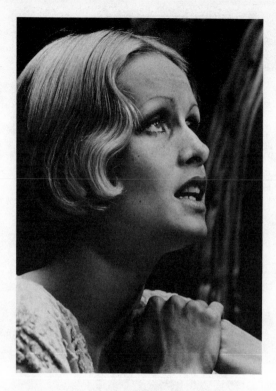

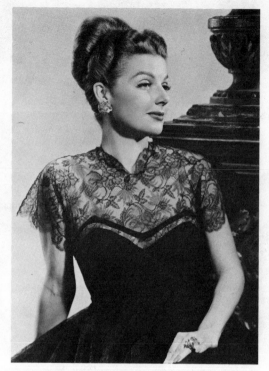

38

37

This former beauty contest winner has proven her acting ability in many motion pictures. She starred in a successful TV series, *Police Woman*.

1. *Angeline Brown.*   2. *Joni Bass Brown.*
3. *Amy Sandler.*

In the sixties she was one of the most-discussed models in the world. Her thin figure was the basis of many stories and was featured on many magazine covers. She appeared in the films *The Boy Friend* and *The Blues Brothers*.

1. *Leslie Hornby.*   2. *Liz Greenberg.*
3. *Janet Radeck.*

39

She was known as "The Oomph Girl" and was a favorite of GIs during World War II. She went from beauty-contest winner to stardom in Hollywood.

1. *Cheryl Anaheim.*
2. *Clara Lou Sheridan.*
3. *Annabelle Sheridan.*

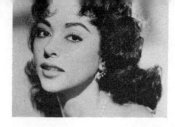

40

This Puerto Rican actress and dancer won an Academy Award for her stellar performance in *West Side Story*. She appears on the stage and TV and in nightclubs between films.

1. *Megan O'Neill.*
2. *Rosita Dolores Alverio.*
3. *Rita y Alvarez.*

41

This beautiful French actress began as a model. She was a leading lady in many international films, captivating audiences with her acting ability and beautiful long legs.

1. *Germaine Lefebvre.*
2. *Arlene Capucine.*
3. *Barbara Carmody.*

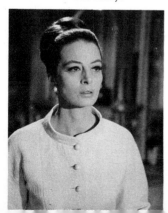

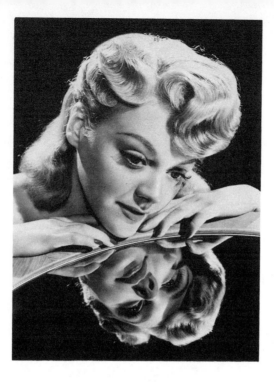

42

She was a beautiful American leading lady in the forties who will be remembered for her role in *Romance on the High Seas*.

1. *Leslie Howard-Brooks.*
2. *Lulu Brookfield.*
3. *Leslie Gettman.*

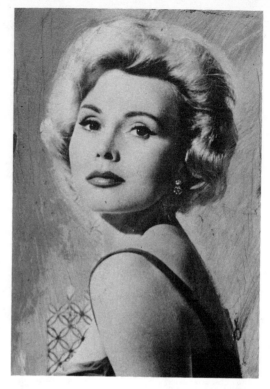

43

She's an exotic international leading lady who was voted "Miss Hungary." She appears infrequently on television and has made several good films in Hollywood. Her speaking style is inimitable.

1. *Gabor Shari.* 2. *Shari Lewis.*
3. *Sari Gabor.*

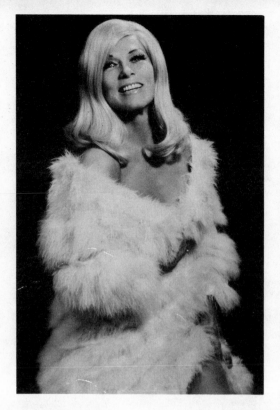

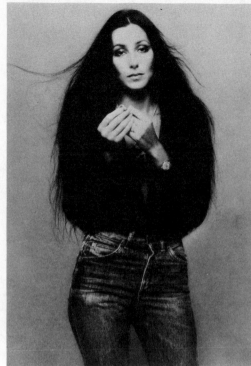

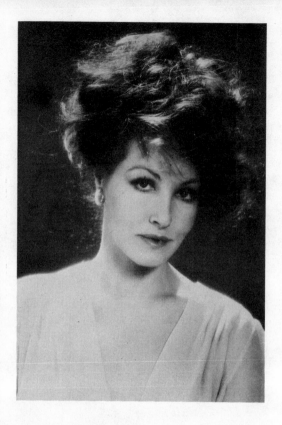

44

This beauteous French actress became a leading lady in Hollywood from 1947. She also appeared on the stage in musical comedies.

1. *Denise Kramer.*   2. *Denise Billecard.*
3. *Danielle Darcelline.*

45

Here's a long-legged, talented singing star whose flair for unusual dresses and attire has made her a real sex symbol. At one time her show was a TV highlight. She has also acted on the Broadway stage.

1. *Charlene Carmody.*   2. *Carol LaDessiere.*
3. *Cherilyn LaPiere.*

46

This statuesque Swedish star captivated movie- and play-goers with her beauty and acting ability.

1. *Julia Newmeyer.*   2. *Ethel Winant.*
3. *Yvonne Demery.*

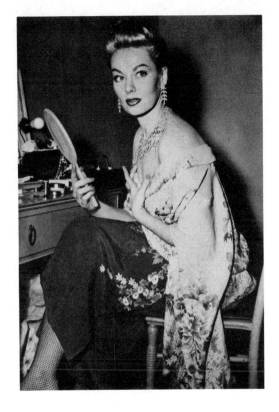

47

One of America's most beautiful ecdysiasts (strippers), who was under contract to Universal Studios and made several films.

1. *Marie Van Schaak.*   2. *Celia Brown.*
3. *Jane Langford.*

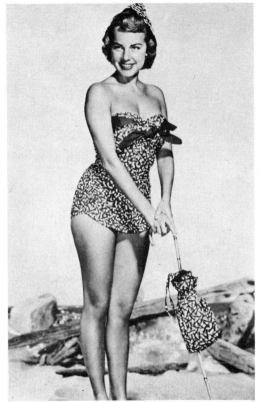

48

She was a child model and appeared in films from infancy. She later was a leading lady, much to the delight of moviegoers everywhere.

1. *Lily Bridges.*   2. *Helen Koford.*
3. *Georgine Seraphine.*

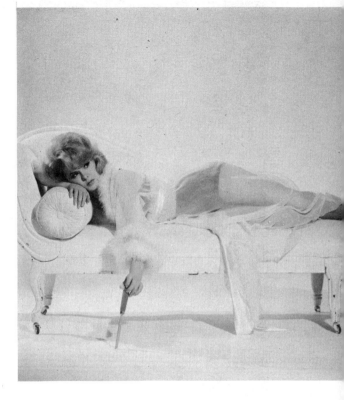

49

She was a former child performer and the daughter of a popular bandleader. She became a luscious leading lady in minor films.

1. *Holly Hollis.*   2. *Molly Lampert.*
3. *Davenie Johanna Heatherton.*

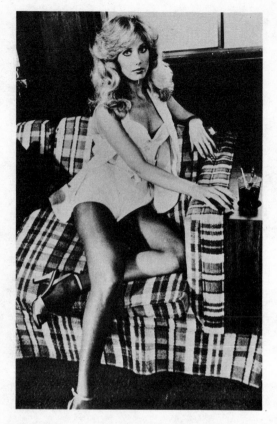

50

This scintillating blond actress appeared in soap operas and achieved stardom in the TV series *Flamingo Road*.

1. *Patty McCormick.*   2. *Patsy McClenny.*
3. *Mimi Grunberg.*

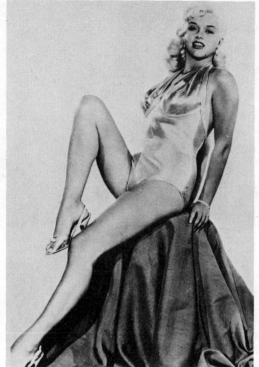

51

One critic called her "Britain's most glamorous export." She made her American film debut in *I Married a Woman*, which co-starred George Gobel. She was married to TV's Richard Dawson.

1. *Maria Matlaga.*   2. *Diana Fluck.*
3. *Diane Ossinger.*

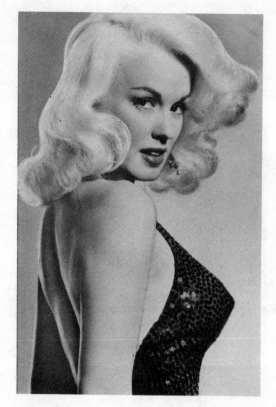

52

Here's a real blond bombshell of the silver screen. As a leading lady in American films, she attracted thousands of moviegoers.

1. *Joan Lucille Olander.*
2. *Mamie Vandenberg.*
3. *Natalie Jacobson.*

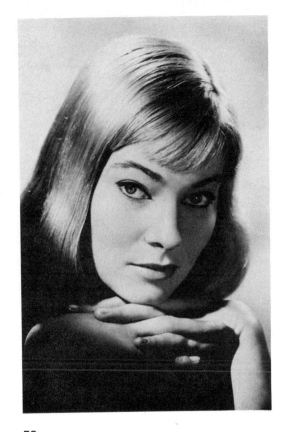

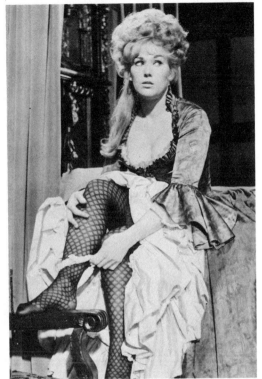

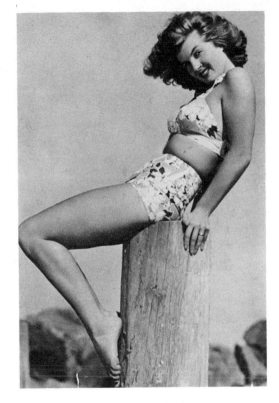

53

This beautiful Swedish actress achieved her success in the remake of *Blue Angel*, which originally starred Marlene Dietrich.

1. *Maybritt Wilkens.*   2. *Susan Denison.*
3. *Leslie Dilley.*

54

This beautiful American actress had her name changed because the studio thought of grooming her as a possible rival to Marilyn Monroe.

1. *Kim Evans.*   2. *Marilyn Bernheimer.*
3. *Marilyn Novak.*

55

A French leading lady, this statuesque blonde had a mildly successful career in Hollywood during the early fifties.

1. *Lauren Kramer.*   2. *Corinne Dibos.*
3. *Sandra Rich.*

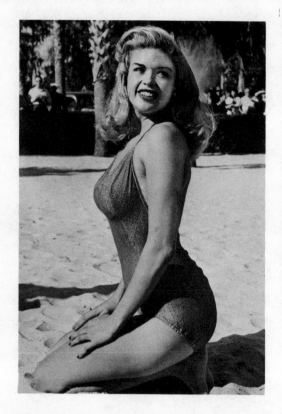

56

This buxom sex symbol played "dumb blonde" roles, but was an experienced comedienne and fine actress until her untimely death in a car accident.

1. *Vera Jane Palmer.*   2. *Joan Mansfield.*
3. *Joan Brannigan.*

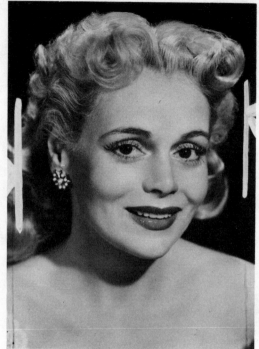

57

She was once called "The Body," due to her imposing proportions. Starting as a model, she sang with Tommy Dorsey's orchestra and went on to Hollywood to find fame as *My Friend Irma.*

1. *Marie Frye.*   2. *Sandy Diamond.*
3. *Katherine Elizabeth White.*

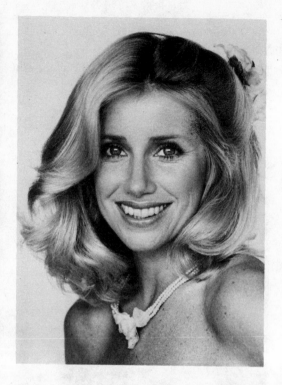

58

An American actress who achieved national acclaim for her "dumb blonde" role in TV's *Three's a Crowd.* She is also a talented singer-dancer and appears in fashionable clubs.

1. *Sherry Lansing.*   2. *Suzanne Mahoney.*
3. *Betty Buckley.*

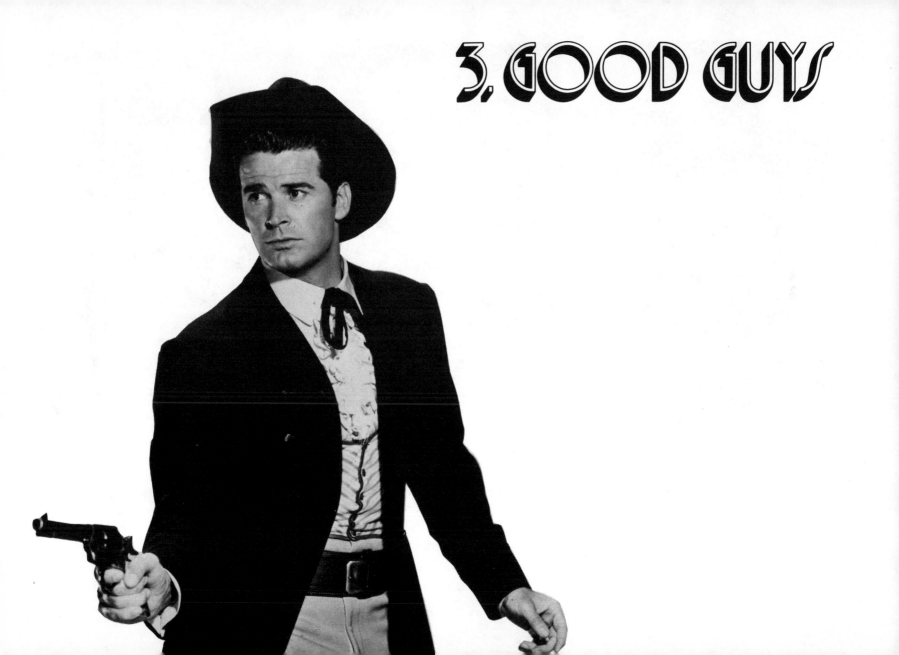

3. GOOD GUYS

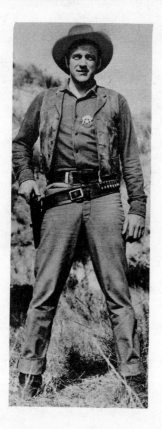

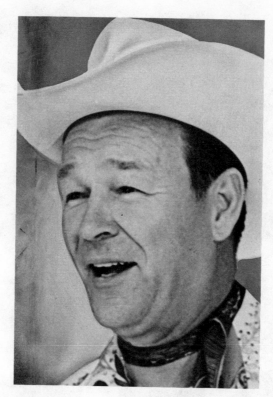

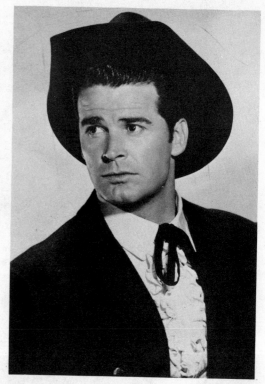

59

A giant of a man, 6 feet 6 inches tall, who drifted into films from advertising. He created the role of "Marshall Dillon" in the successful TV series *Gunsmoke* and appeared in *McClaine's Law*.

1. *James R. Gaines.*   2. *James Aurness.*
3. *Joe Indelli.*

60

He is a famous singing cowboy who was usually seen with his popular horse "Trigger." He began singing with "The Sons of the Pioneers," who later appeared in his many Hollywood films. He was also a popular TV favorite.

1. *Roy Levin.*   2. *Leonard Slye.*
3. *Roger Williams.*

61

He's an amiable, good-looking American leading man who is well known for his TV commercials for a camera company. He had a successful TV series, *Maverick*.

1. *James Baumgarner.*
2. *James J. O'Malley.*
3. *Joseph Tirinato.*

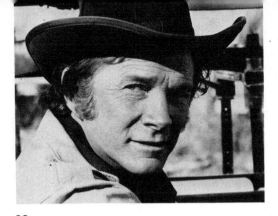

62

This handsome leading man is the brother of Dana Andrews, the popular American actor. He appears frequently on TV.

1. *Dick Steeves.*   2. *Larry Gershman.*
3. *William Andrews.*

63

After a successful naval career, he became a leading man in films. His TV series, *Wild Bill Hickock*, was a hit.

1. *Robert Moseley.*   2. *Robert A. Parsons.*
2. *Edward A. Montanus.*

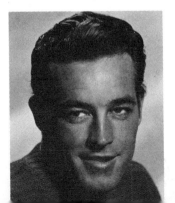

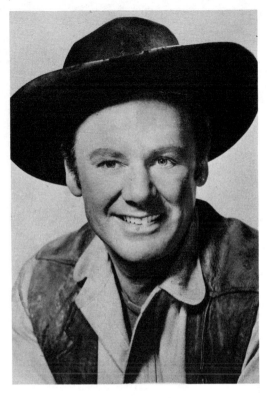

64

He is an American leading man who has proved to be a great talent on the stage, too. He was exceptional in *Miracle in the Rain*.

1. *Charles Van Johnson.*   2. *Phil Corper.*
3. *Colman Andrews.*

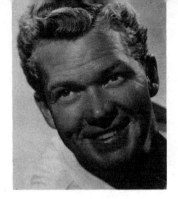

65

This handsome, rugged he-man of the silver screen was known as "Kit Carson." He is married to Barbara Hale, known as "Della Street" on the TV series *Perry Mason*.

1. *Win Baker.*   2. *Richard B. Stolley.*
3. *William Katt.*

66

This genial American leading man was former boxer and stunt man. He was married to Dinah Shore.

1. *Stewart Tilger.*   2. *George M. Letz.*
3. *Dick Pryce.*

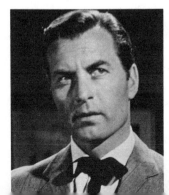

39

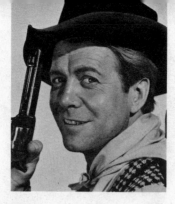

67

This long-legged dancer-singer was a success in many musical films and on the stage. He is a versatile director, too.

1. *Jon Mutter.*   2. *George V. Smith.*
3. *Eugene Berg.*

68

He was a cheerful American leading man who began as an extra in films after some vaudeville experience with his parents.

1. *Edward "Bud" Flanagan.*
2. *Rocco Paoletta.*   3. *Steve Minasian.*

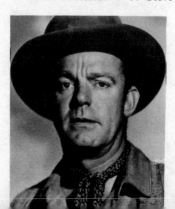

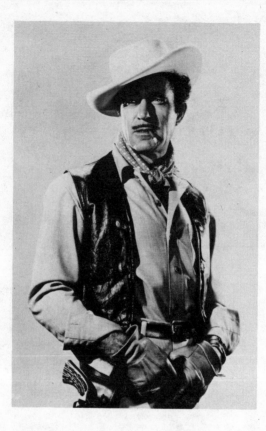

69

He was a leading Mexican actor who trained as a bullfighter. He became a popular hit in Hollywood in the mid-twenties and thereafter.

1. *Bill Newman.*   2. *Ivan Bender.*
3. *Luis Antonio de Alonso.*

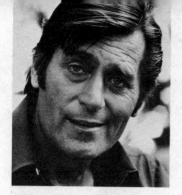

70

He's a giant-sized American leading man and former cowboy hero of TV's *Cheyenne*. He has made Hollywood films.

1. *Norman E. Walker.*   2. *William Miller.*
3. *Noah Sallop.*

71

This handsome actor-director starred on TV in *Bonanza* and became famous as the director of the successful TV series *The Little House on the Prairie.*

1. *Michael Orowitz.*   2. *Thomas Bender.*
3. *Michael Landers.*

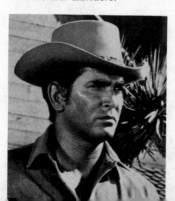

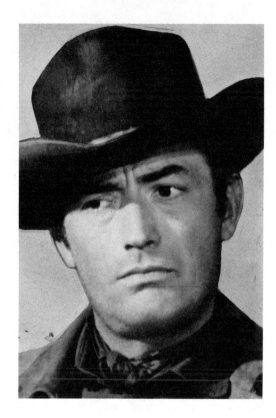

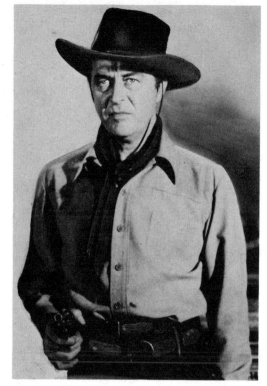

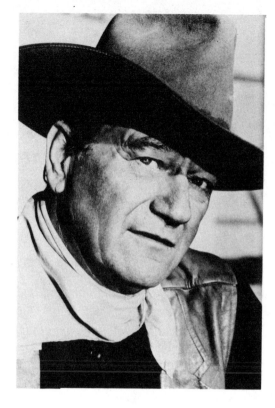

72

This durable and likeable American leading man had a great deal of stage experience before sudden success in Hollywood. He won an Oscar for his performance in *To Kill a Mockingbird*.

1. *Gregory Plank.*   2. *Brian S. McNiff.*
3. *Eldred G. Peck.*

73

This handsome Welsh-born actor carved a niche for himself in Hollywood and won an Oscar for his role in *Lost Weekend*.

1. *Ray Mann.*
2. *Reginald Truscott-Jones.*
3. *Millard Manton.*

74

He was a tough, genial, and inimitable American leading man of action films who became one of the best known and most successful Hollywood actors.

1. *Marion M. Morrison.*   2. *Wayne Johnson.*
3. *John Wainwright.*

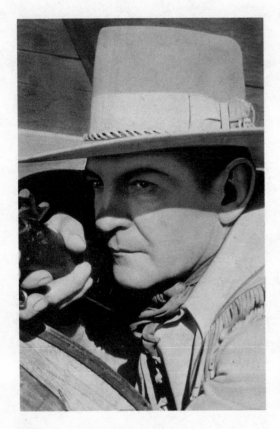

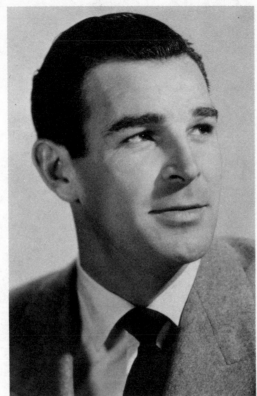

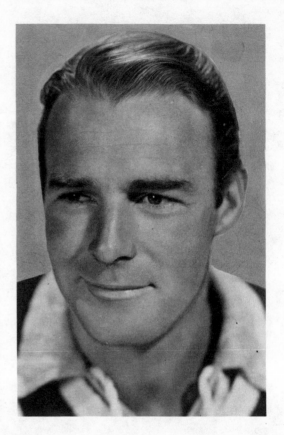

75

This fine western actor lost his life in the ill-fated Cocoanut Grove fire in Boston in 1942. He made many successful Hollywood films.

1. *Dean Jones.*   2. *Charles Jones.*
3. *Bob Darling.*

76

This rugged Canadian star came to Hollywood where he appeared in many succesful films. He was once a stand-in for actor Fred MacMurray.

1. *Nathan Cox.*   2. *Steve Pettepit.*
3. *Robert J. Landry.*

77

This rugged Hollywood actor played many "cowboy" roles after much stage experience.

1. *John Hollister.*
2. *George Randolph Crane.*
3. *Scott Randolph.*

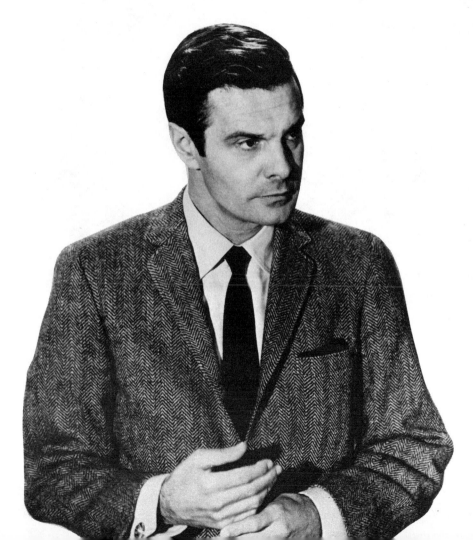

4. LEADING MEN

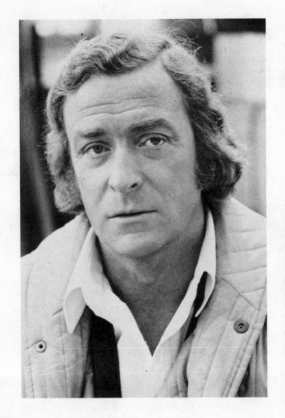

78

A British leading man with an effective, mild manner who is hailed in America as a major star. His performance in *Sleuth* will long be remembered.

1. *Maurice Micklewhite.*   2. *Jess Caine.*
3. *Joseph Sargon.*

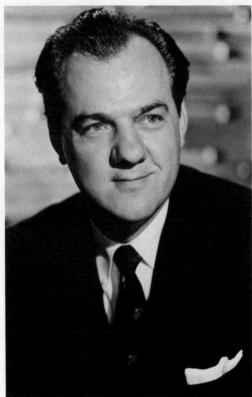

79

An American actor who appears on TV advertising *that* credit card and who made a big hit in TV's *Streets of San Francisco.*

1. *Carl Rudnick.*   2. *Megan O'Neill.*
3. *Malden Sekulovich.*

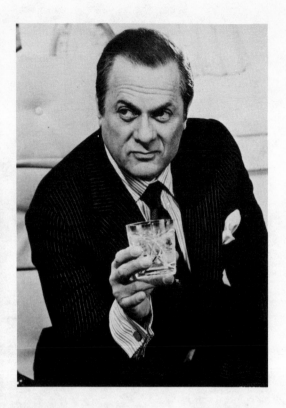

80

A fine American actor whose name was changed by a producer. He became a leading man and appeared in scores of films and is seen on TV.

1. *Bernard Schwartz.*
2. *William W. Schwartz.*
3. *Tony Capodilupo.*

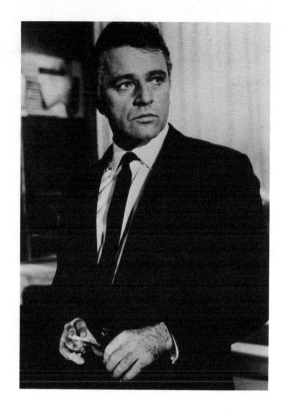

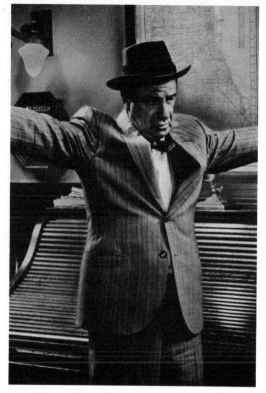

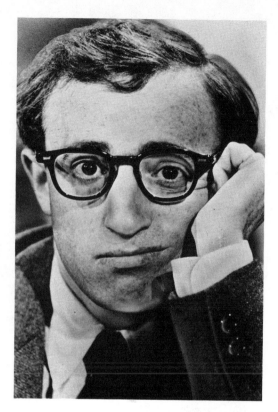

81

A brilliant Welsh actor who was married to Elizabeth Taylor. He captivated American audiences on stage and screen.

1. *Richard Jenkins.*   2. *Ken Page.*
3. *Robert Henshaw.*

82

An American character actor with a flare for comedy which has made him a big star.

1. *Walter Matuschanskayasky.*
2. *Anthony Morris.*
3. *Fred Silverman.*

83

He's a bespectacled American comedian and light playwright who makes chaotic films catering to a sophisticated audience.

1. *Robert Henshaw.*
2. *Allen Stewart Konigsberg.*
3. *Walter Staab.*

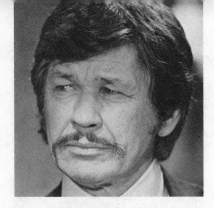

84

He's a sombre-looking, deep-featured actor who plays varied roles, from villainous to sturdily heroic.

1. *Charles Buchinski.*   2. *Charles Walters.*
3. *Bob Frank.*

85

A rugged, handsome leading man in Hollywood films, who had the unusual attraction of prematurely gray hair. He was spectacular as "Cochise" in *Broken Arrow*.

1. *Ira Grossel.*   2. *Jefferson Hall.*
3. *Chandler Peerce.*

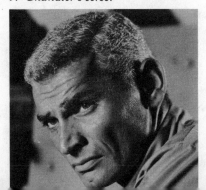

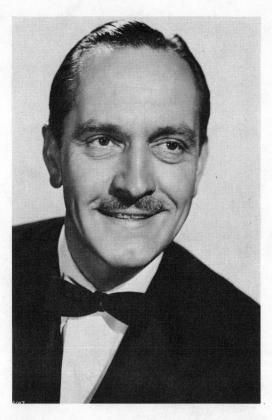

86

He won an Oscar in *The Best Years of Our Lives*. He was one of America's most respected stage and screen actors, whose performances projected integrity and intelligence at all times.

1. *Frederick Brodney.*   2. *Fred Hadge.*
3. *Frederick McIntyre Bickel.*

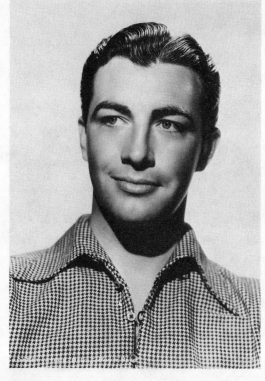

87

An American actor whose handsome appearance and deep voice made him a popular star and leading man. His real name was one of the glories of our culture.

1. *John Matlaga.*
2. *Spangler Arlington Brugh.*
3. *Tony DeMauro.*

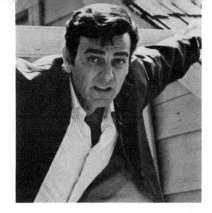

88

Formerly known as "Touch" Connors, this handsome actor achieved renown on his TV series *Mannix* and *Today's FBI*.

1. *Robert F. Bradley.* 2. *R. Dlement Darling.*
3. *Kreker Ohanian.*

89

An American leading man with considerable stage and radio experience, known as "the man who invented the telephone," from his role in *The Story of Alexander Graham Bell*.

1. *Don M. DeHart, Jr.* 2. *Paul Gerken.*
3. *Dominic Felix Amici.*

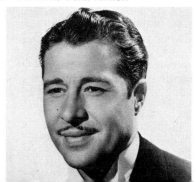

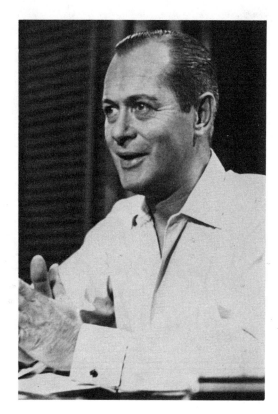

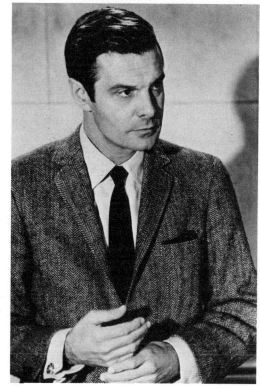

90

He was a smooth, handsome, and brilliant American leading man who became a director, then forsook acting for politics.

1. *Joe Fortini.* 2. *Mark Robinson.*
3. *Henry Montgomery, Jr.*

91

He's a smooth French leading man who made many Hollywood films and appears on TV and the stage.

1. *Jean Mayer.* 2. *Louis Gendre.*
3. *Louis Fagioli.*

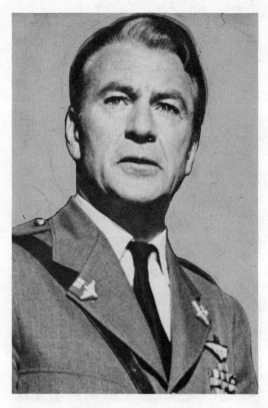

92

This slow-speaking, deep-thinking American leading man had a long and enduring career as a Hollywood star. He won an Oscar for *Sergeant York*.

1. *Dick Cooper.*   2. *Ron Cayo.*
3. *Frank J. Cooper.*

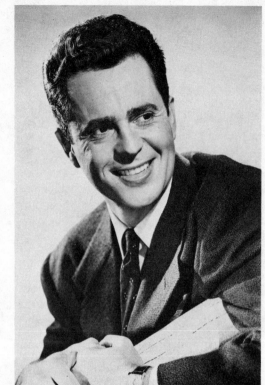

93

This American leading man scored heavily in the film *The Jolson Story*, playing the role of the great entertainer Al Jolson.

1. *Don Taylor.*   2. *Samuel Klausman.*
3. *Same Dame.*

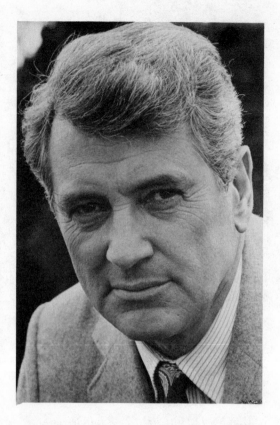

94

This giant-sized American leading man moved from western films to light comedies and starred in a successful TV series, *McMillan and Wife*.

1. *Norm Prescott.*   2. *Bill Marlow.*
3. *Roy Sherer.*

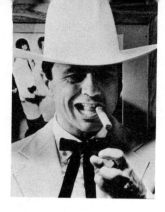

95

He began as a child movie actor and became a big hit on TV in a series, *Baretta*.

1. *Fred Pierce.*   2. *Richard Ballinger.*
3. *Michael Gubitosi.*

96

This young, handsome actor has appeared in many American films, notably *Apocalypse Now*, and on TV in *The Execution of Private Slovik*.

1. *Martin Sheehan.*   2. *Ramon Estevez.*
3. *Bud Greenspan.*

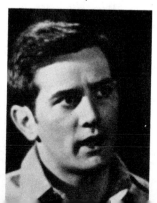

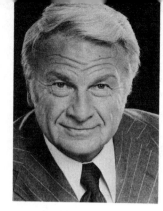

97

This popular American character actor began as a radio and stage performer and had a big TV series, *Green Acres*. He appears on the big screen, too.

1. *Mike Dann.*   2. *Eddie A. Heimberger.*
3. *Ted Herbert.*

98

He was in local politics before becoming a Hollywood actor. He had a gravel voice and beefy physique.

1. *Aldo Da Re.*   2. *Stanley Colman.*
3. *Ray Adlow.*

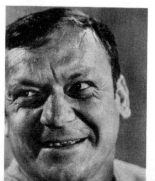

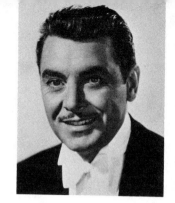

99

He was an Irish-born American actor who was in films in Hollywood from 1930 to the early fifties. He appeared as a leading man, co-starring with the likes of Bette Davis and Myrna Loy, with great distinction.

1. *George Cashman.*   2. *George B. Nolan.*
3. *Fred MacNeill.*

100

This handsome American leading man was an athletic actor who became a star with his first major Hollywood film, *Hurricane*, with Dorothy Lamour.

1. *John Hallberg.*   2. *John Halburton.*
3. *Charles Locher.*

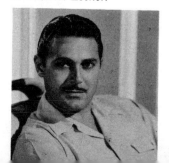

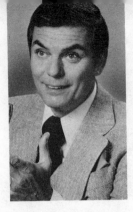

101

He's a very talented comedian and has hosted TV's *Hollywood Squares* for many seasons. He is a favorite in Las Vegas, Reno, and Lake Tahoe clubs.

1. *Peter De Reow.*   2. *Marshall Peterson.*
3. *Pierre LaCock.*

102

A former radio announcer with a rich voice who went to Hollywood and became a leading man in many films.

1. *Hugh Hipple.*   2. *Hugh Downs.*
3. *George Gloss.*

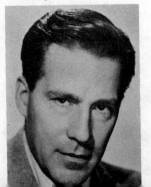

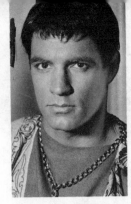

103

This handsome he-man was a Hollywood leading man who also starred on TV in *Destry* and *Convoy.*

1. *Stan Jablonski.*   2. *John Golenor.*
3. *Mike Donovan.*

104

This tall, talented character actor and leading man with premature white hair starred in *Mission Impossible* on TV.

1. *Peter Town Watson.*   2. *Peter Aurness.*
3. *Michael Dukakis.*

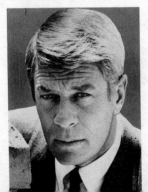

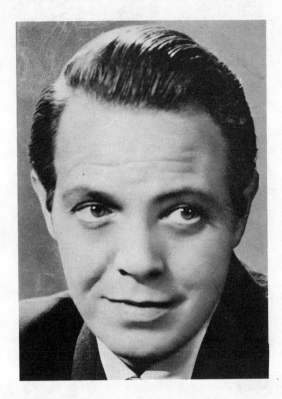

105

He was a mild-mannered, South African-born leading man with stage experience. He was married to actress Ida Lupino, and made many Hollywood films as a leading man.

1. *David Town Watson.*
2. *Seafield Grant.*
3. *Louis Woodward.*

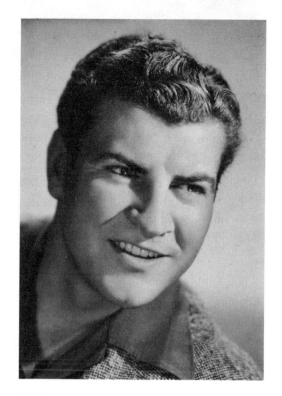

106

This American movie star became a theatre star of great vitality, especially with his role in *The Music Man*, which he also re-created on the screen.

1. *Robert P. Messervey.*
2. *John F. Collins.*
3. *Barney Frank.*

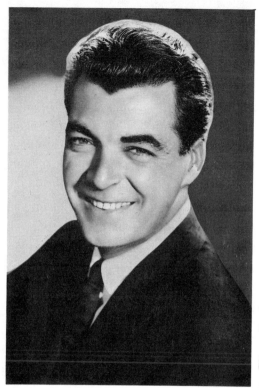

107

He is an amiable American leading man who made many action films in the fifties. On TV he starred in *The Texan*.

1. *Francis Timothy Durgin.*
2. *Tom Brokaw.*
3. *Robert Radnitz.*

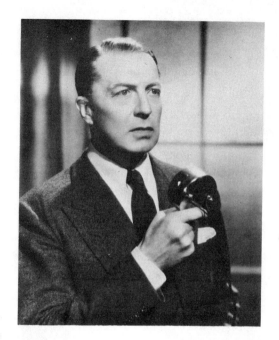

108

He was a distinguished British leading man of stage and screen for over forty years, playing the "perfect gentleman" or occasional "caddish" roles in Hollywood films in the thirties and forties.

1. *Clifford Brook.*   2. *David Dortort.*
3. *Cliff Brookfield.*

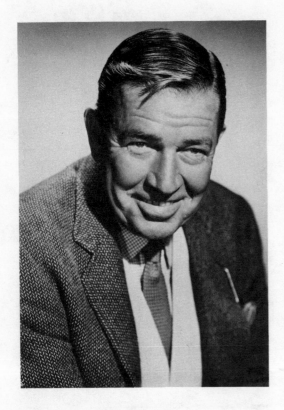

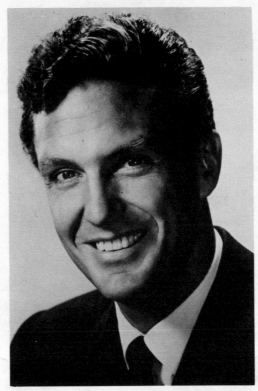

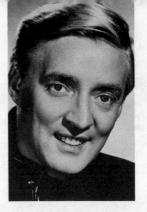

111

He's a fine Austrian leading man with international screen and stage credits. He was outstanding in *Ship of Fools*.

1. *Oscar Brodney.*
2. *Josef Bschliessmayer.*   3. *Oscar Spinner.*

112

He's a fine American actor who has excelled on stage and screen since the late forties. He was seen on the TV series *House Call*.

1. *Wayne McKeekan.*
2. *H. Weller Keever.*   3. *Peter Lucas.*

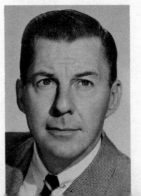

109

He was a square-jawed American film hero of many action-adventure films in the thirties. He was in the original *King Kong*.

1. *Etienne Pelissier de Bujac.*
2. *Rick Kinsman.*
3. *Paul Tsongas.*

110

He's a personable, cold-eyed American leading man who made it big as a star of the TV series *The Untouchables* and *The Name of the Game*.

1. *Robert Modini.*
2. *Robert Stackpole.*
3. *Rufus Sachs.*

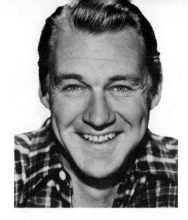

113

This tall, good-looking and good-humored actor was a leading man in Hollywood from the early forties. He was a Yale graduate.

1. *Bowen Charleston Tufts III.*
2. *Sonny Jurgenson.*   3. *Sonny Fox.*

114

This British comedian started in show business in 1935 as "Mot Snevets." He is identified by the gap between his front teeth.

1. *Thomas Terry Hoar-Stevens.*
2. *Tom Clark.*   3. *Tom Sullivan.*

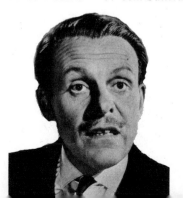

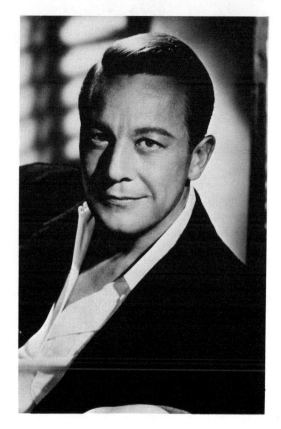

115

This handsome, blond American actor was married to singer-actress Jeanette Macdonald. He was on the stage from childhood.

1. *Gene Rayburn.*   2. *Raymond Guion.*
3. *Eugene Massey.*

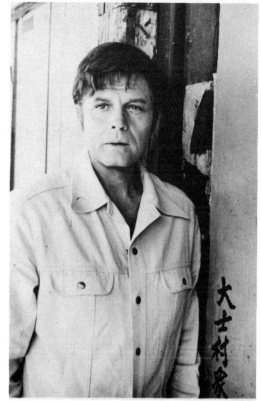

116

This fine American actor became a legend when he appeared in his TV series *Hawaii Five-O.* As a craggy-faced hero he found his niche in TV.

1. *John Joseph Ryan.*   2. *Jackson Lordly.*
3. *John Larssen.*

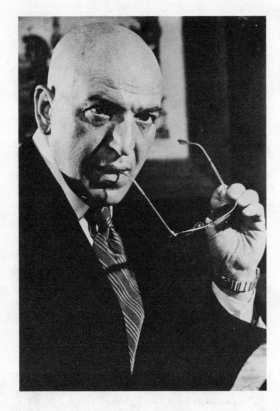

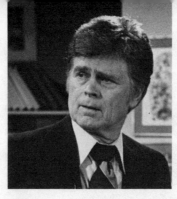

118

This stocky actor appeared in many American films as a leading man and is adept in stage plays. He appeared on TV in *My Favorite Husband* and *Hudson's Bay*.

1. *Robert Neilson.* 2. *Baryy Lynnfield.*
3. *Nelson O'Hara.*

119

A rugged, he-man type actor with a gaunt appearance who has made many memorable American films. He has much stage experience and hosted a TV series, *Believe It or Not*.

1. *Walter Palahnuik, Jr.* 2. *Irv Rothman.*
3. *Dan Capozzi.*

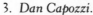

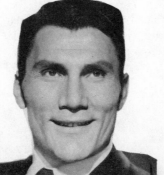

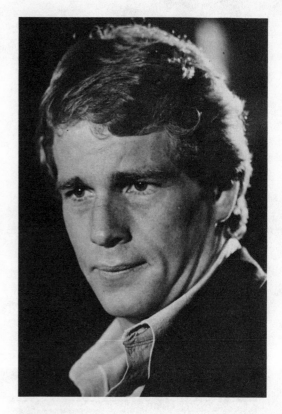

117

This Greek-American character actor made many films and became a big hit in his TV series *Kojak*.

1. *Seville Talas.*
2. *Aristotle Savalas.*
3. *Dean Anagnos.*

120

He was a bland juvenile actor who made it big in the TV series *Peyton Place* and scored heavily in many motion pictures.

1. *Bryan O'Neill.*
2. *Patrick R. O'Neal.*
3. *Neal Ryan.*

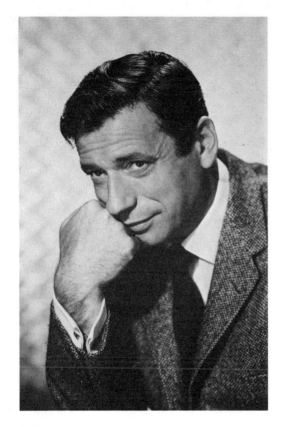

121

This French actor-singer starred with Marilyn Monroe in *Let's Make Love*. He married French actress Simone Signoret.

1. *Francois Phouf.*   2. *Ivo Levi.*
3. *Emil Suave.*

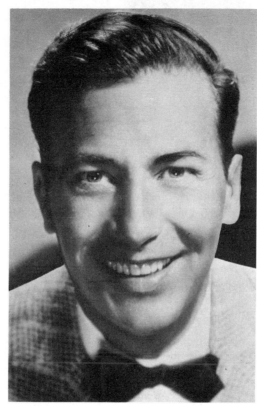

122

This handsome American leading man was a love-interest in many films, beginning with *Four Daughters*.

1. *Jeffre Wheller.*   2. *Ragnar Lind.*
3. *Jefferson Lindbrook.*

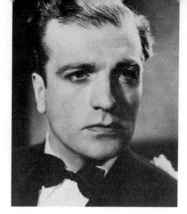

123

This handsome British star became a successful character actor after music-hall and stage experience.

1. *John Lowe.*   2. *John Carson.*
3. *John Ackerman.*

124

He was a handsome leading man in American films during the thirties. Women catered to his many whims on the screen.

1. *Michael LoPresti.*
2. *Joseph Kenneth Shovlin.*   3. *Joseph Sholkin.*

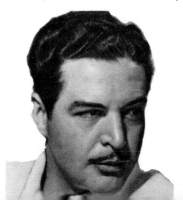

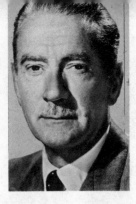

125

He was a former dancer and stage star in musical comedies. He became a leading American character actor playing waspish, middle-aged roles.

1. *Clifton Holmes.*   2. *Cliff Webster.*
3. *Webb Parmalee Hollenbeck.*

126

This American leading man had a pleasantly bemused air. He won an Oscar in *They Shoot Horses Don't They?*

1. *Stanley Kayne.*   2. *Bryon Barr.*
3. *Gregory Young.*

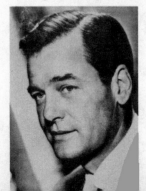

127

Here is an early photo of this American leading man, who guided the destinies of actress Bo Derek early in her career. He was one of the handsomest men on the screen.

1. *Derek Harris.*   2. *Bob Pecora.*
3. *John Dirckson.*

128

He was referred to as a "beefcake hero" of the sixties, and made many a teenager swoon as a romantic screen hero.

1. *Al Katz.*   2. *Merle Johnson.*
3. *Sherm Feller.*

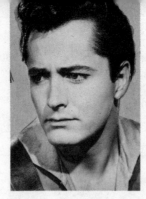

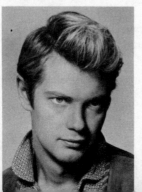

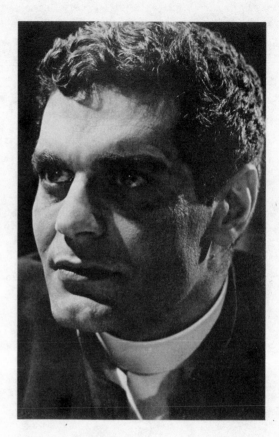

129

This Egyptian leading man is a romantic Hollywood star. He was magnificent in *Dr. Zhivago*, *Lawrence of Arabia* and other films.

1. *Omar Harrow.*   2. *Michel Shalhouz.*
3. *Sharo Omar-Fassi.*

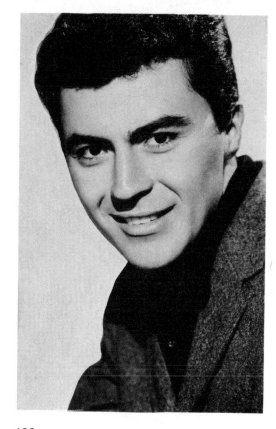

130

Another handsome American leading man who seemed to have special appeal for a vast younger audience. He made a TV series, *Time Tunnel*.

1. *Anthony Athanas.* 2. *James Droney.*
3. *James Ercolani.*

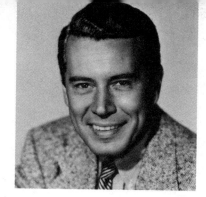

131

He's a smooth American actor who was heard as "The Voice" on TV's popular series, *Charley's Angels,* and is a leading man on the stage and in films. He also stars in TV's *Dynasty*.

1. *John Powers.* 2. *John Freund.*
3. *John F. Collins.*

132

A former successful model, he graduated to leading man roles in Hollywood films. He had a TV series called *The Bold Ones*.

1. *Carmen Orrico.* 2. *John Reed.*
3. *John Sackson.*

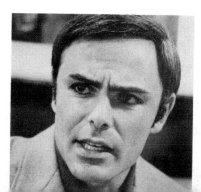

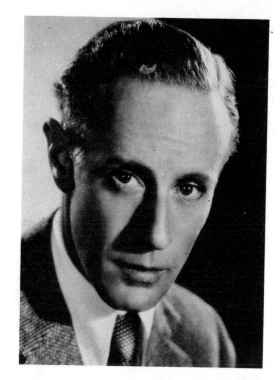

133

This distinguished British actor was of Hungarian origin. His image was that of an intellectual who had only to ignore women to be idolized by them. He was a huge success in American films, but mysteriously came up "missing" in an airplane accident during World War II.

1. *Lazlo Steiner.* 2. *Rex Reed.*
3. *Leslie Hore.*

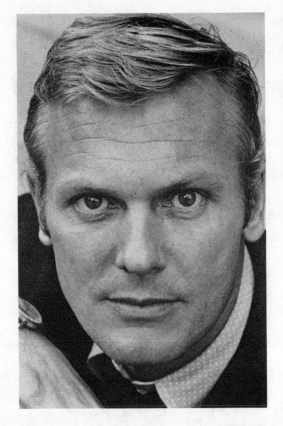

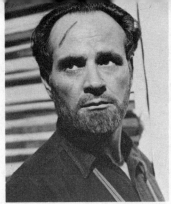

135

This Hungarian actor was a big star in the silent films and early "talkies." He appeared in many Cecil B. DeMille movies.

1. *Mihaly Varkonyi.*   2. *Dick O'Connell.*
3. *Mikail Victor.*

136

This American stage actor made several good films, including Hitchcock's *Rope* and *The Corn Is Green*.

1. *Donald Rogers.*   2. *Joseph Westheimer.*
3. *John Thompson.*

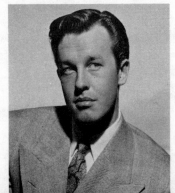

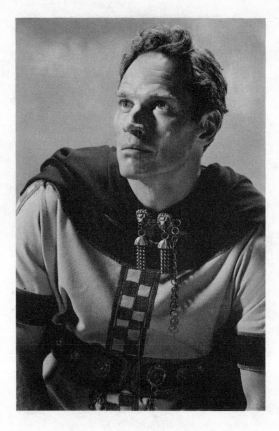

134

A teenage idol during the fifties and an athletic American leading man who is still active in the movies, his most recent being *Polyester*.

1. *Arthur Gelien.*   2. *Bill Glazer.*
3. *Billy Baxter.*

137

This stalwart American leading man played in many biblical and medieval epics on the screen. He has vast stage experience, also.

1. *Charles Hiss.*   2. *Carlton Hessian.*
3. *Charlton Carter.*

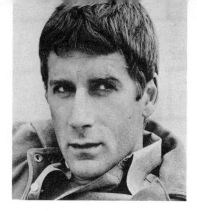

138

This Italian-American leading man scored big in films, especially *Synanon*.

1. *Alexander Viespi.*   2. *Alex Schmootz.*
3. *Alec Trician.*

139

This American leading man became a Latin lover in the Rudolph Valentino mould in the twenties. He took his name from a well-known cigar at the time.

1. *Jacob Kranz.*   2. *Richard Carton.*
3. *Dick Carson.*

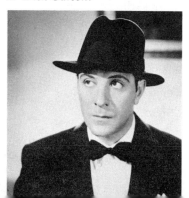

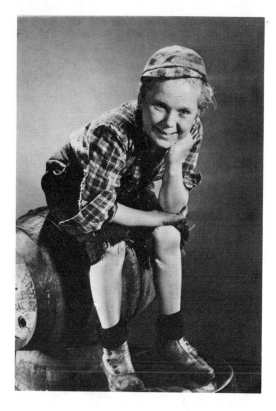

140

This "little tough guy" American child actor scored as "Skippy" in early films. He later became a skilled motion picture actor and powerful TV executive.

1. *John Bigelow.*   2. *Jackie Adams.*
3. *Kevin White.*

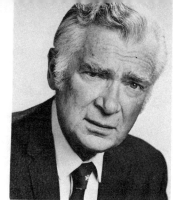

141

This fine American actor-dancer-singer was a huge success with his sister in musical comedies. His later, greater success was on TV in *The Beverly Hillbillies* and *Barnaby Jones*.

1. *William E. Hood.*
2. *Christian Rudolf Ebsen.*   3. *David Sendler.*

142

He's a dapper French actor of stage and screen who has been in films since 1930. He made many films in Hollywood.

1. *Claude Franc-Nohain.*
2. *Claude Bowles.*   3. *Claude Huppè.*

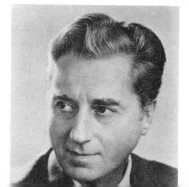

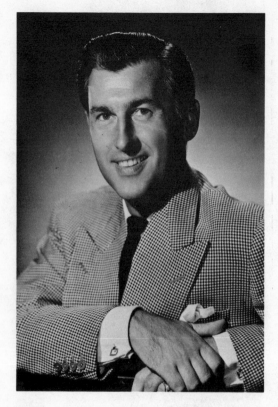

143

This handsome British leading man came to Hollywood but had to change his real name because someone else was using it. He was married to Jean Simmons.

1. *Stuart Steinberg.*   2. *James Stewart.*
3. *James Craig.*

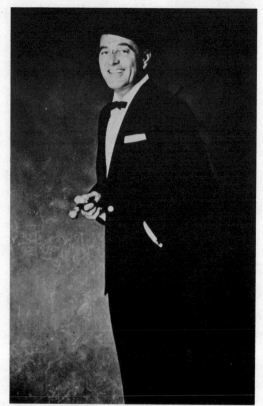

144

This former cabaret singer and leading man in American films became a star of motion pictures after years of traveling with dance bands.

1. *Alfred Morris.*   2. *Tony D'Abruzzi.*
3. *Anthony Sousa.*

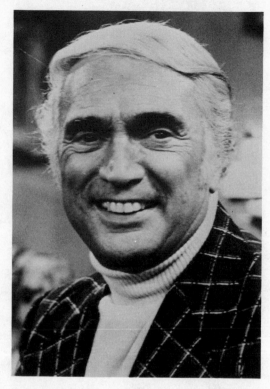

145

This fine American leading man came from the stage and has much experience in radio. His son is actor Alan Alda. He gave a fine interpretation of George Gershwin in the film *Rhapsody in Blue.*

1. *Robert Charm.*   2. *Alan Brooks.*
3. *Alphonso d'Abruzzo.*

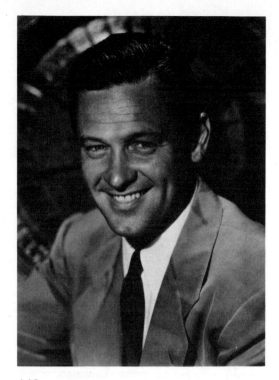

146

This handsome leading man won an Oscar for his sterling role in *Stalag 17*. He hardly ever gave a bad performance, as evidenced by such hit films as *Golden Boy, Sunset Boulevard, Born Yesterday, The Bridge on the River Kwai*, and others.

1. *William Beedle, Jr.*   2. *Bill Fitch.*
3. *Tim Jarrel.*

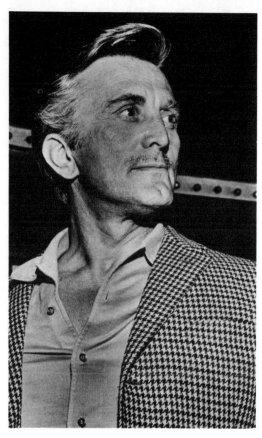

147

An American leading man and a fine actor who plays intelligent heroes in films of many kinds.

1. *Allan Angoff.*   2. *Douglas Kirsten.*
3. *Issur Danielovitch Demsky.*

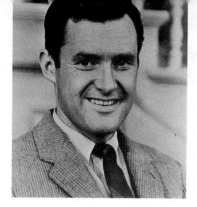

148

A very funny fellow who appears frequently on TV. He started as a magician and chose the weirdest name he could think of.

1. *Orson Wellington.*   2. *Dallas Burrows.*
3. *Arthur Hamilton.*

149

A craggy American character actor of the fifties and the sixties, he was an all-purposeful leading man. He was notable in *Airport 69*.

1. *Emmett Evan Heflin.*   2. *Neil Evans.*
3. *Roger Youman.*

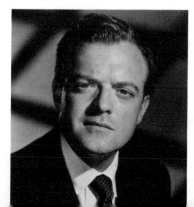

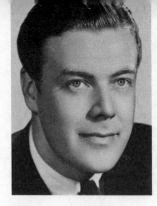

150

He was a tennis pro who appeared on the stage in *Johnny Belinda* and in many Hollywood films.

1. *William Manchester.*   2. *Willard Parkinson.*
3. *Worster Van Eps.*

151

He was a star athlete long before gaining fame on the screen. He was a member of the U.S. Olympic team, held the shot put championship in the U.S.A., and was an all-American football star. He was a "Tarzan" and a leading man in other Hollywood films.

1. *Bruce McCabe.*   2. *Herman Brix.*
3. *Victor Kendall.*

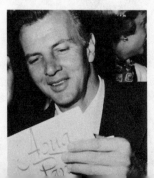

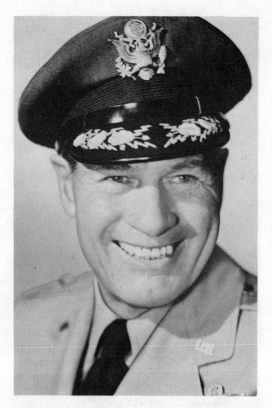

152

A handsome American actor who scored as a hero-type in *Wings*, one of the first Oscar-winning films.

1. *Cornelius van Mattemore.*
2. *Richard D. Zanuck.*
3. *Frederic Steinkamp.*

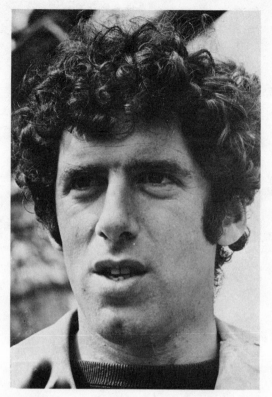

153

An American actor who was a big hit in the seventies and is still a favorite of many moviegoers and TV viewers. He was once married to Barbra Streisand.

1. *Eliot Aronson.*   2. *Elliot Goldstein.*
3. *Eliot Nussbaum.*

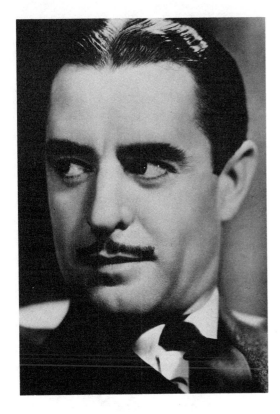

154

An American leading man of the twenties who came from a theatrical family. Unfortunately, he found that his voice was less dashing than his looks when the "talkies" began.

1. *John Pringle.*   2. *John Knotts.*
3. *Larry Whiteside.*

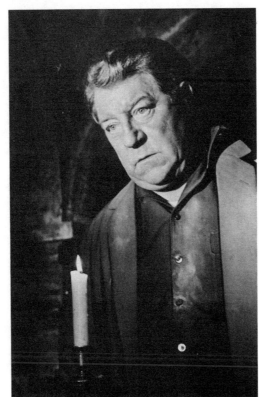

155

A great French actor who distinguished himself as an international star from the early thirties.

1. *Alexis Moncourge.*
2. *Paul J. Reale.*
3. *Jean Ganbin.*

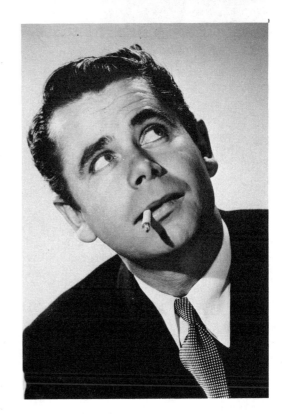

156

This Canadian-born star of many American films has continued his stardom from a young leading man to more mature hero-roles, with great success.

1. *Gwyllyn Ford.*   2. *Ford Sterling.*
3. *Glenn Blivitz.*

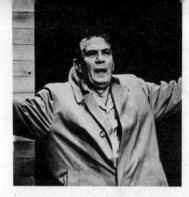

157

He became an international star and the idol of millions of Americans after a brilliant career in Australia. He was awarded the Academy Award, posthumously, for his role in *Network*.

1. *William Ingle-Finch.* 2. *Peter Potter.*
3. *Peter Flincheim.*

158

He's a British-born comic actor who achieved success in an American TV series, *Mr. Ed*, the adventures of a talking horse.

1. *Angus Young.* 2. *Alan Ladd, Jr.*
3. *Hal Elias.*

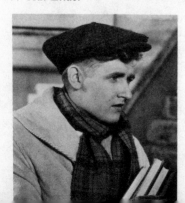

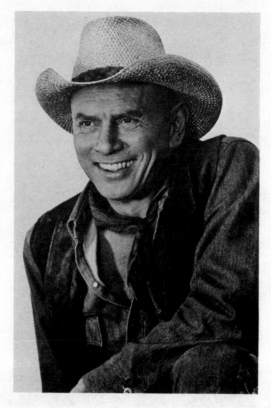

159

This strikingly bald international star of somewhat mysterious background achieved immortality as the King in *The King and I*, both on the stage and on the screen.

1. *Don Hall.* 2. *Bryan Yulbrunner.*
3. *Tadje Kahn, Jr.*

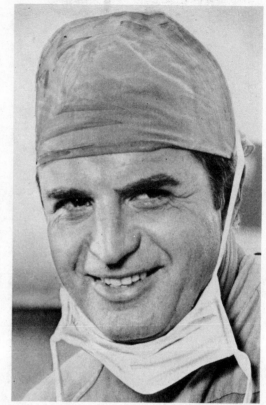

160

He's a tough, brash type of leading man who made his mark as "Dr. Casey" in the TV series, *Ben Casey*, during the mid-sixties.

1. *Vincent E. Zoimo* 2. *Chuck Young.*
3. *Larry Mahoney.*

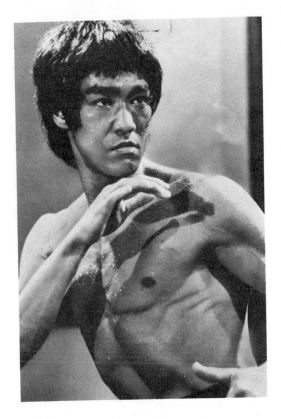

161

A talented writer, actor, and director, he became famous for his martial arts films, such as *Game of Death*.

1. *Li Jun Fan.* 2. *T. Hoe.*
3. *Pat Sazuki.*

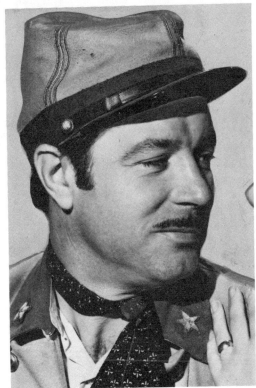

162

This American leading man usually played the good-natured but tough outdoor type. His best role was in *All That Money Can Buy*, in which he played the Faust character.

1. *Craig James.* 2. *James Meador.*
3. *Jamie Dineen.*

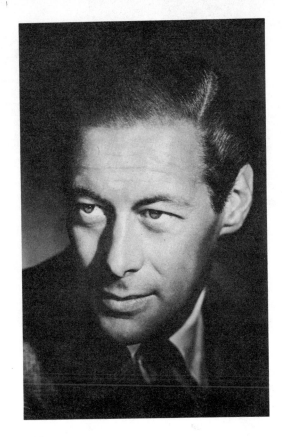

163

This debonair British actor won an Oscar for his stellar performance in *My Fair Lady*, in which he had acted on the stage, too.

1. *Al Krivin.* 2. *Ben Bradley.*
3. *Reginald Carey Harrison.*

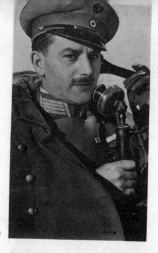

164

This German actor was in British films from the mid-thirties. He played in many distinguished films, such as *The Red Shoes*.

1. *Adolf Wohlbruck.* 2. *Adolph Shickelgruber.*
3. *Mike Weinblatt.*

165

This handsome, rugged actor is a fine singer who made many Hollywood films, and also starred in *Dallas* on TV.

1. *Howard M. Spiess.* 2. *Harold Keel.*
3. *Harold O. Kinsman.*

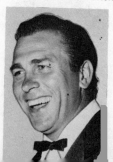

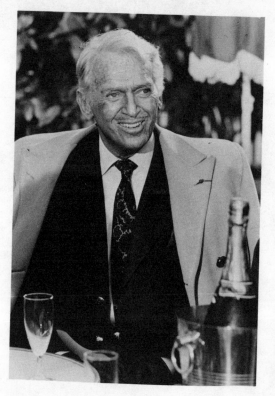

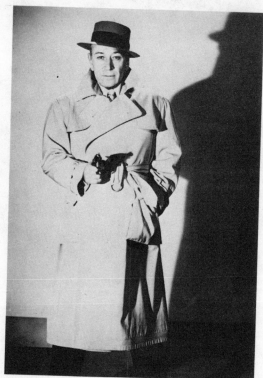

166

This debonair, handsome Hollywood actor spent much time in Britain, and made innumerable TV films.

1. *Anthony Thomopoulos.*
2. *Douglas Elton Ulman, Jr.*
3. *Norm Nathan.*

167

He catapulted to stardom while flipping a coin in the film *Scarface*. He made scores of films as a sinister companion of gangsters. He was formerly a professional ballroom dancer.

1. *Pat Flynn* 2. *George Ranft.*
3. *George Back.*

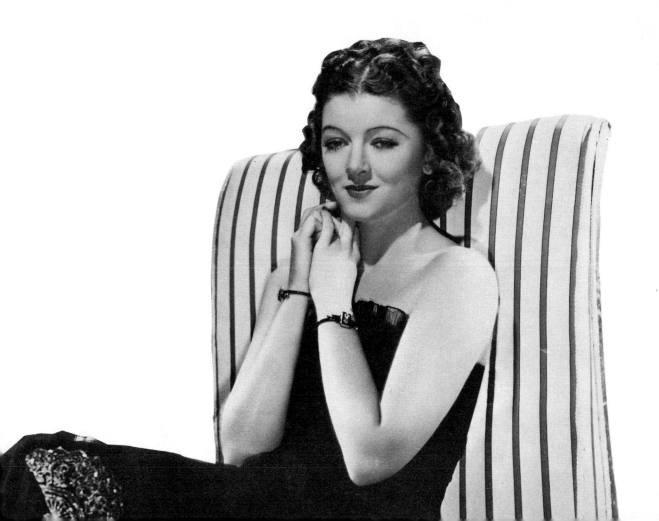

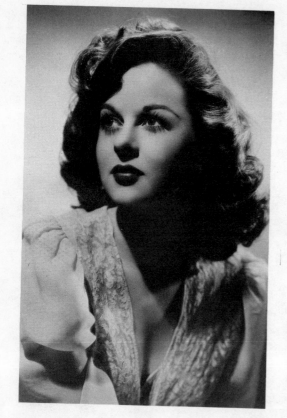

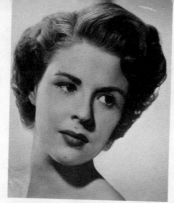

169

She was a former child actress who matured into leading lady roles in many Hollywood films.

1. *Mary Ellen Powers.* 2. *M. Allah-Prost.*
3. *Martha Oregon.*

170

This vivacious, long-legged actress is married to actor Richard Benjamin. She went right from college to Hollywood as a leading lady.

1. *Paula Pentagon.* 2. *Paula Perkoff.*
3. *Paula Ragusa.*

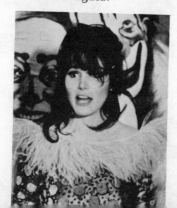

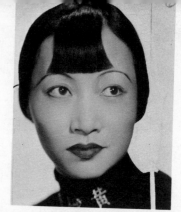

171

This beautiful oriental actress was popular during the silent film days and during the early thirties. Her performances were scintillating.

1. *Sew Leong Kwa.* 2. *Wong Liu Tsong.*
3. *Siew-Wah Ho.*

172

She is a pleasing actress who got her training in American radio, TV, and films. She is a well-known cosmetics firm executive.

1. *Pauline Berger.* 2. *Paula Bergenheim.*
3. *Nellie Burgin.*

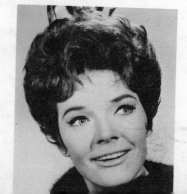

168

This Academy Award winner for her roles in *I'll Cry Tomorrow* and *I Want to Live* was a vivacious leading lady in scores of American films.

1. *Edythe Marriner.* 2. *Susan Browle.*
3. *Sue Ann Hayes.*

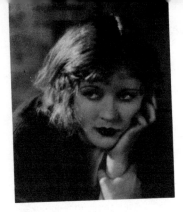

173

This pert Anglo-French actress was a leading lady in Hollywood films, especially during the silent era. She influenced hair style among American women.

1. *Marie Bickford Dunn.* 2. *Mary Proctor.*
3. *Elaine Prescott.*

174

With a brief stage experience this lovely actress went to Hollywood and became a leading lady in many films. She appeared on TV in a series, *Janet Dean, Registered Nurse.*

1. *Ella Rainstorm.* 2. *Ella Raubes.*
3. *Ella Foible.*

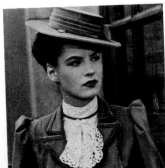

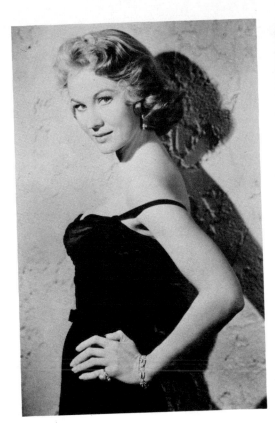

175

A beautiful American actress who flourished in the truest tradition of "peaches-and-cream" roles.

1. *Ginny Mahoney.* 2. *Virginia Jones.*
3. *Wendy Moger.*

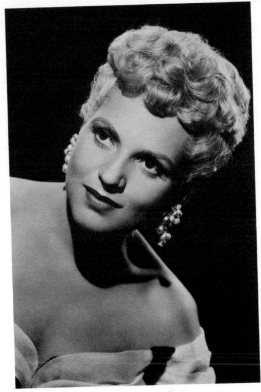

176

This beautiful-but-dumb-acting star of Hollywood films won an Academy Award for her role in *Born Yesterday.* She was a superior comedienne.

1. *Judith Tuvim.* 2. *Judy Proskauser.*
3. *Judith Purim.*

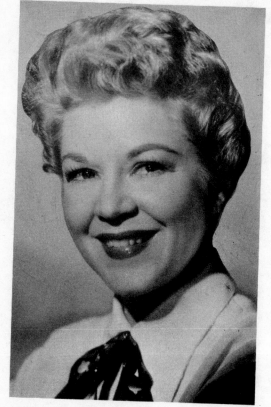

177

She was a great character actress in Hollywood who appeared in many films and achieved critical acclaim. She was a child stage actress.

1. *Claire Wemlinger.*   2. *Claire Tremor.*
3. *Clare Windsor.*

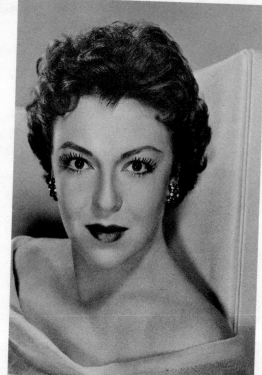

178

She was a Spanish dancer and actress who appeared on the American stage and screen. She married actor Eddie Albert.

1. *Margo d'Alfonso.*
2. *Maria Boldao y Castilla.*
3. *Margo Antonelli.*

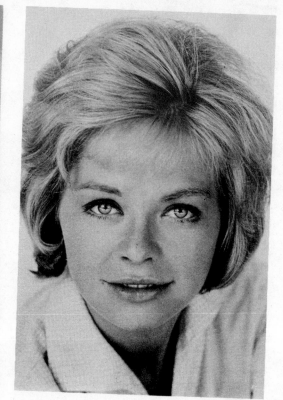

179

This beautiful British star made many American films and is in great demand as a leading lady.

1. *Susannah Yolande Fletcher.*
2. *Fay Kanin.*
3. *Jean Firstenberg.*

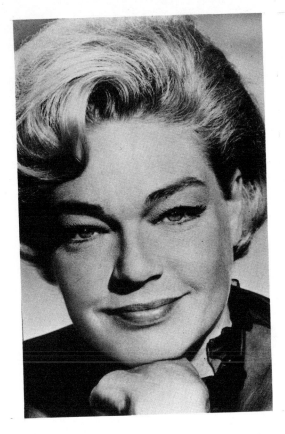

180

This distinguished French actress won an Oscar for her role in *Room at the Top*. She married Yves Montand.

1. *Adrienne LaRussa.*   2. *Jeanine Basinger.*
3. *Simone-Henriette Kaminker.*

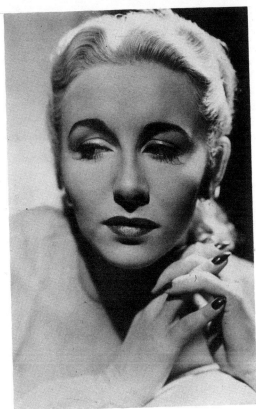

181

This lovely Czech actress was a former skating champion. She married the boss of Republic Studios, Herbert Yates, and became its star.

1. *Vera Hruba.*   2. *Hubra Veraraalston.*
3. *Frances Marie Rizzo.*

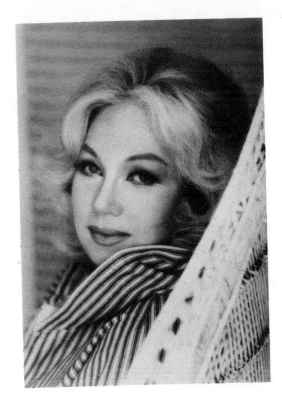

182

This lovely American actress had much stage experience. She went on to become a fine comedienne and leading lady. She starred in *Private Secretary* and *The Ann Southern Show* on TV.

1. *Priscilla Barnes.*   2. *Harriette Lake.*
3. Annmarie Peet.

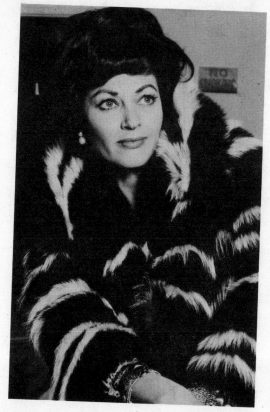

183

She was born in Canada and became a leading lady in Hollywood. She was a big star during the forties.

1. *Zelma Ardon.*   2. *Peggy Middleton.*
3. *Yvonne Vanicola.*

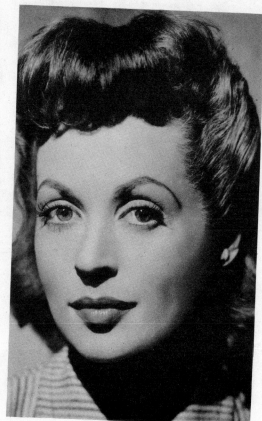

184

She was on the stage since her childhood days in Austria, and in films since a teenager.

1. *Lillian Palmerston.*   2. *Lily Palm.*
3. *Maria Lilli Peiser.*

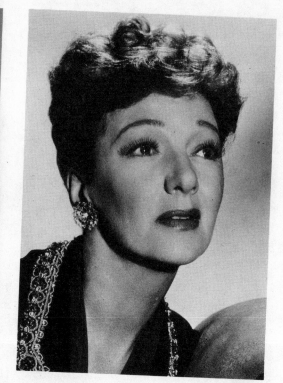

185

She was one of the stage-screen's greatest talents. As a British actress and singer she starred in several Noel Coward plays. She was excellent in the Hollywood movie *The Glass Menagerie.*

1. *Gertrude Lowell.*
2. *Alexandre Lawrence-Klasen.*
3. *Gert von Ferde.*

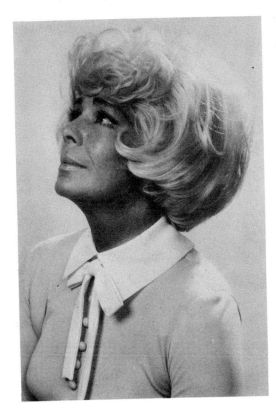

186

A blond, bouncy American leading lady of many singing/dancing light entertainments of the forties and fifties. She was superb in *The Miracle of Morgan's Creek*.

1. *Betty van Fleet.*   2. *Betty Hooten.*
3. *Betty Jane Thornburg.*

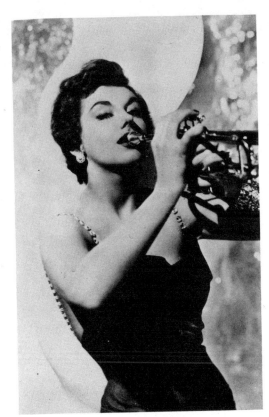

187

She was a vivacious, stylish British actress and leading lady of the fifties. She was married to actor Rex Harrison.

1. *Justine McCarthy.*   2. *Kay Kardon.*
3. *Katherine Crandall.*

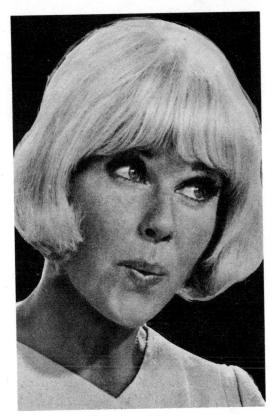

188

A beautiful actress who portrayed "the girl next door" in many of her box-office hits. She began as a singer with Les Brown's orchestra.

1. *Doris Kappelhoff.*   2. *Dorothy Daye.*
3. *Doris Deyton.*

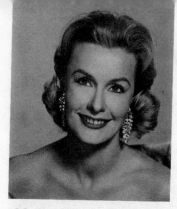

189

She's a beautiful, leading socialite who made many films. She is married to actor Cliff Robertson.

1. *Natalie Colman.*
2. *Nedenia Hutton Rumbough.*
3. *Denna Murrow.*

190

This glamorous leading lady has appeared opposite some of Hollywood's greatest stars.

1. *Natalie Jacobson.*
2. *Karen Blanche Ziegler.*   3. *Blanche Urban.*

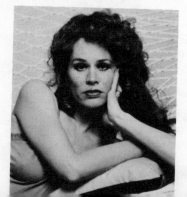

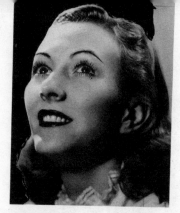

191

She was a glamorous leading lady in Hollywood during the thirties.

1. *Mildred Linton.*   2. *Karen Moseley.*
3. *Clara Muir-Lee.*

192

This American leading lady made her big hit in the TV series *Hart to Hart*, co-starring with Robert Wagner.

1. *Wilhelmina Protell.*
2. *Stefania Federkiewicz.*
3. *Staphanie Power-Tule.*

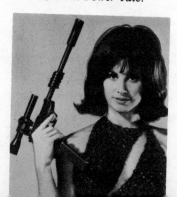

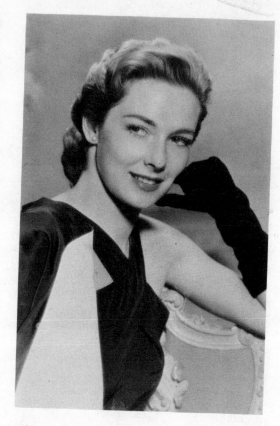

193

This beautiful Hollywood actress came to movies from TV. She scored big in Hitchcock's thriller *Psycho*.

1. *Vera Ralston.* 2. *Vera Hogan.*
3. *Vera Walker-Mile.*

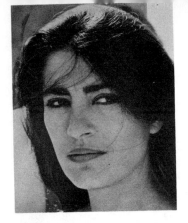

194

She is a Greek stage actress who has made films abroad and in the U.S., to great acclaim.

1. *Irene Patrukus.* 2. *Irene Lelekos.*
3. *Irene Gapoulos.*

195

She is a sultry, beautiful French actress who scored heavily in American and Eruopean films, especially *A Man and a Woman.*

1. *Nanouk Ovthenorth.*
2. *Annette Chason.*
3. *Françoise Sorya Dreyfus.*

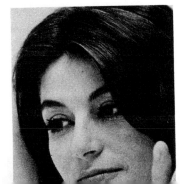

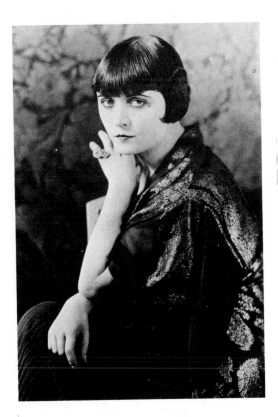

196

This popular Polish-born leading lady went to Hollywood and was a popular star until sound came in.

1. *Pearl Chandoeicz.*
2. *Paula Nibrbenwiecs.*
3. *Appolonia Chalupek.*

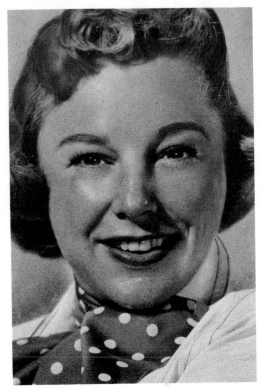

197

This lovely, husky-voiced American Leading lady was equally ready with a tear or a smile. She was married to actor Dick Powell. She also appeared on TV in her own series.

1. *Evirginia Lewiecki.*   2.*Ella Geisman.*
3. *June Arlington.*

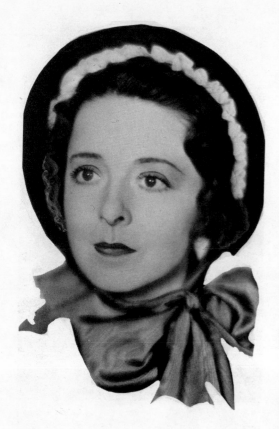

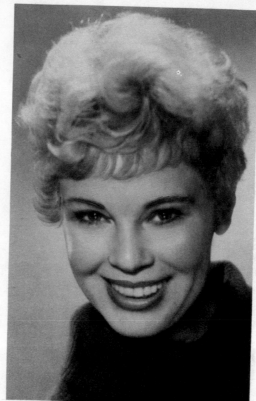

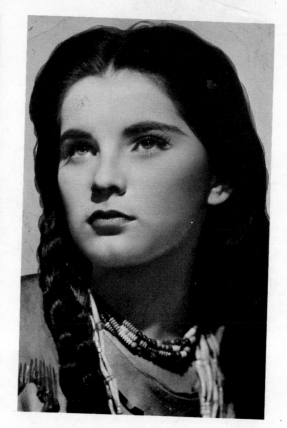

198

A great actress of the silent era of films, she made her first film in 1917 and starred in *The Scarlet Letter*.

1. *Stefanie More.*   2. *Carla Morrison.*
3. *Kathleen Morrison.*

199

A fine stage actress who has made many notable American films. She also appears frequently on television as a panelist.

1. *Patricia Brumbeck.*   2. *Betsy Ross.*
3. *Betty Buffington.*

200

This beautiful American actress played ingenues and graduated to leading lady roles in the fifties.

1. *Debra Lee.*   2. *Debralee Griffin.*
3. *Deborah Parquette.*

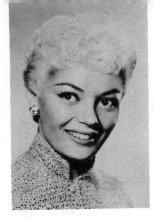

201

She was a former dancer and became a favorite leading lady in American films, usually playing a blond seductress.

1. *Dawn Bethel.*   2. *Cheri Nauson.*
3. *Shari Northern.*

202

This beautiful leading lady appears in many Hollywood films and starred on TV in *The Jimmy Stewart Show.*

1. *Julia Adamson.*   2. *Betty May Adams.*
3. *Judy Allison.*

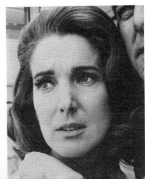

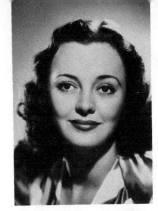

203

She was an American leading lady of the early forties. She gave an excellent performance in *Stage Door.*

1. *Anne Leader.*   2. *Antoinette Lees.*
3. *Leah Anson.*

204

A beautiful actress who appeared in American films and is adept as a radio/TV comedienne. She appeared in her own TV series, *The Cara Williams Show.*

1. *Clarisse Williamson.*   2. *Carla Winters.*
3. *Bernice Kamiat.*

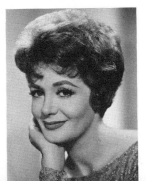

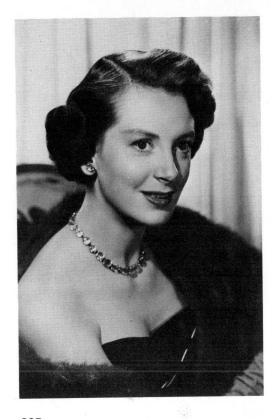

205

This elegant British actress played many dramatic roles in Hollywood, notable in *The King and I, The Night of the Iguana, From Here to Eternity,* and others.

1. *Deborah Kerr-Trimmer.*
2. *Debbie Snow.*   3. *Debra Carlson.*

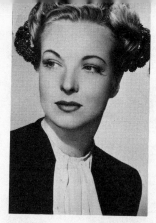

206

This statuesque blond beauty was a Hollywood leading lady during the forties.

1. *Hilda Brooks.*   2. *Beatrice Peterson.*
3. *Helen Bucher.*

207

This beautiful French leading lady made a few American movies and married Errol Flynn.

1. *Lily Schnee.*   2. *Lillian Damask.*
3. *Lilliane Carre.*

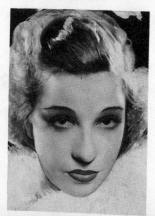

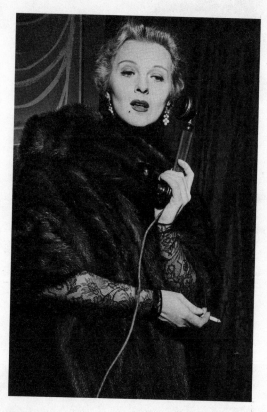

208

No relation to actor Raymond Massey, she was born in Hungary and came to Hollywood where she made films and became a singer and TV star.

1. *Regina Gluss.*   2. *June Foray.*
3. *Ilona Hajmassy.*

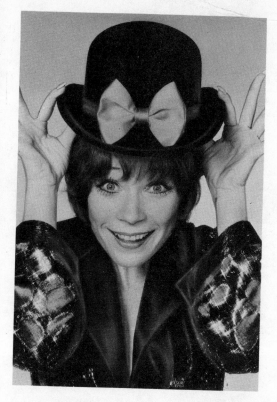

209

This impish, multi-talented singing-dancing actress, made a big hit in *Irma La Douce* and *Sweet Charity*. She is also a best-selling author.

1. *Shirley M. Beaty.*
2. *Elisa Sequin.*
3. *Shirley McClaine.*

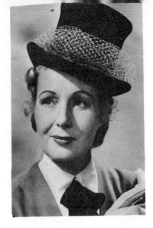

210

This fine English actress enacted roles as a self-confident, smart, wisecracking leading lady.

1. *Gitelle Enoyce Barnes.*   2. *Ginnir Gloss.*
3. *Virginia Bohlin.*

211

She began as a child actress and pianist and developed into a fine, pert, witty American leading lady.

1. *Dolores Loehr.*   2. *Diana Bromberg.*
3. *Diane Lynnfield.*

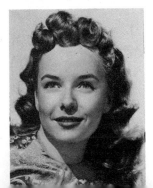

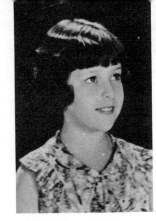

212

She was a brilliant child actress in the thirties who matured into a bright, talented stage actress as she grew older.

1. *Elizabeth Keno.*   2. *Mitzi Halfgaynor.*
3. *Marian Greenhawker.*

213

She was a fine Hollywood Actress and leading lady who married singer-actor Bing Crosby.

1. *Katherine Grandstaff.*
2. *Kathy Bernheimer.*   3. *Cathy Coppersmith.*

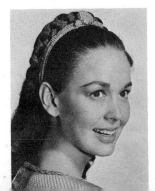

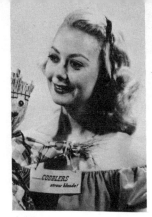

214

This beautiful, luscious Spanish-American dancer played leading lady roles in the forties and fifties.

1. *Adelaide Delgado.*   2. *Adele Krensky.*
3. *Adelaide Maren.*

215

This beautiful Hollywood actress was a leading lady in many successful films, especially *Red River*, with John Wayne.

1. *Doris Jensen.*   2. *Anne Crystal.*
3. *Muriel Bookhalter.*

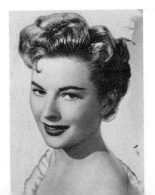

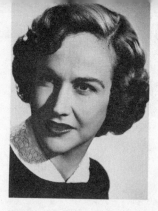

216

A very talented, pert, and dependable Hollywood actress who starred with Marlon Brando in *A Streetcar Named Desire* and appeared in many other films.

1. *Kim Perkins.*   2. *Janet Cole.*
3. *Kimberley Higgins.*

217

This vivacious redhead was one of the reasons that *Guys and Dolls* was such a smash stage and film success.

1. *Vivienne Stapleton.*   2. *Vivian Rasnick.*
3. *Ellen Sandler.*

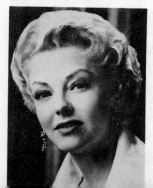

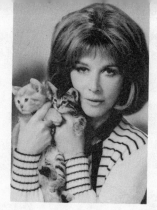

218

This very talented American actress is a dynamic stage performer seen in stellar roles in Hollywood films and on TV. She was excellent in *Shampoo.*

1. *Leah Granville.*   2. *Lee Gruntberger.*
3. *Lyova Rosenthal.*

219

Here's another beautiful French actress who had great stage experience and became a leading lady on the screen.

1. *Micheline Chassagne.*   2. *Michele Lee.*
3. *Michele Presley.*

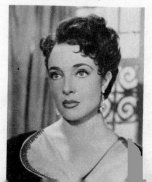

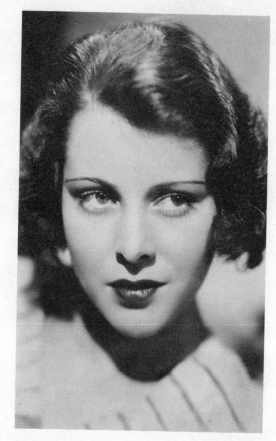

220

A beautiful American film star who married actor Joel McCrea and is still happily married.

1. *Jean Dee.*   2. *Helen Dee.*
3. *Didi Francis.*

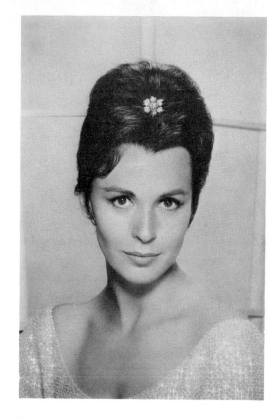

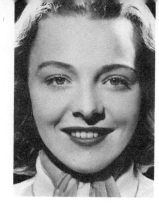

222

She played sympathetic roles in Hollywood films as a leading lady of the late thirties.

1. *Louise Speiss.*   2. *Jane O'Brien.*
3. *Kathi O'Connor.*

223

This talented Hungarian actress was a sensation in international films, and made many American films.

1. *Eve Adamoson.*   2. *Eva Sjöke.*
3. *Evita Batox.*

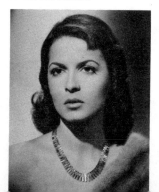

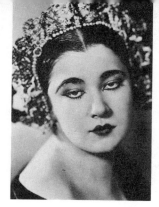

224

A siren in early movies such as *Dr. Jekyll and Mr. Hyde, Blood and Sand,* and *The Ten Commandments.*

1. *Anita Donna Dooley.*   2. *Nita Azzapynn.*
3. *Donna Dretz.*

225

A veteran Warner Bros. Pictures star, born in Englewood, N.J. She appeared in scores of films from RKO and MGM Pictures.

1. *Jean M. Fullerton.*   2. *Jean R. Fulleron.*
3. *Jean A. Fullerton.*

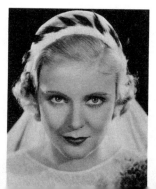

221

This talented British actress came to the screen via the Old Vic and made many prestigious Hollywood films. She was married to actor Rod Steiger.

1. *Clare Bloomington.*   2. *Cara Bloomer.*
3. *Claire Blume.*

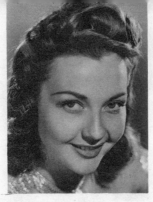

226

This pert American actress often played "the other woman" roles. She began as a chorus girl and rose to good roles in Hollywood films.

1. *Lynn Barry.*   2. *Lyn Loden.*
3. *Marjorie Bitzer.*

227

Her grandfather was General Sir Charles Warren, head of Scotland Yard. She was born in Hong Kong and made many successful films as an American leading lady.

1. *Wendy Blackmer.*   2. *Bari Winston.*
3. *Margaret Wendy Jenkins.*

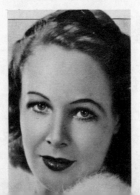

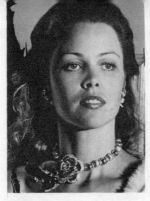

228

This beautiful actress was an accomplished singer. She appeared as the leading lady in *Valentino* in the mid-seventies.

1. *Michele Fulton.*   2. *Holly Howard.*
3. *Holly Michelle Gilliam.*

229

A fine stage and screen actress who achieved stardom as "Edith" in *All in the Family* on TV.

1. *Jeanne Murray.*   2. *Sharon Staples.*
3. *Jean Appleton.*

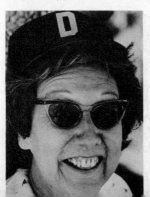

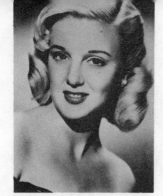

230

This blond actress made many Hollywood films and was notable in *Ace in the Hole*. She made her debut in *Johnny Belinda*, and was married to actor Paul Douglas.

1. *Jane Stirling.*   2. *Jan Silversmith.*
3. *Jane S. Adriance.*

231

She is a fine Hollywood actress with much radio/TV and stage experience. She was a well-known actress during the late forties.

1. *Emily Marie Bertelson.*   2. *Marie Wilson.*
3. *Mary Wilson-Carter.*

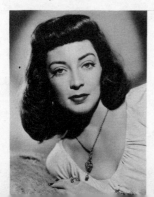

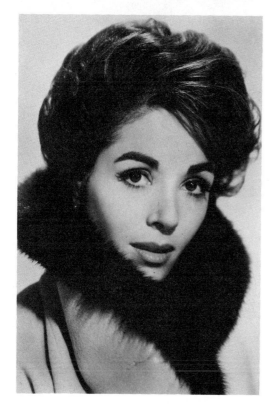

232

This beautiful, enticing British actress made many films in Hollywood. She won acclaim in the original version of *The Invasion of the Body Snatchers*.

1. *Dana Lordly.*   2. *Dagmar Wynter.*
3. *Winnie Darling.*

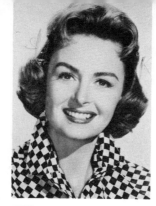

233

This Academy Award winning actress (for her role in *From Here to Eternity*) had a very popular TV show, *The Donna Reed Show*. She won a screen test after winning a beauty contest in college.

1. *Donna Mullenger.*   2. *Donna Reid.*
3. *Donna Redfield.*

234

This fine actress's father is a famous composer and her brother is a renowned movie director.

1. *Talia Rose Coppola.*   2. *Shirley Talia.*
3. *Rose T. Cukor.*

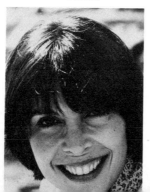

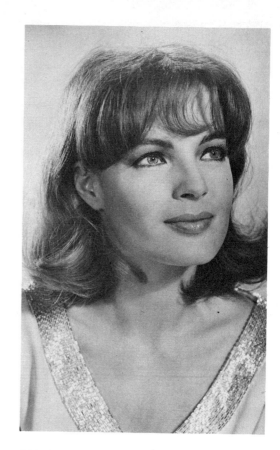

235

This beautiful Austrian-born actress became a favorite international movie star.

1. *Rona Snyder.*   2. *Romella Schneid.*
3. *Rosemarie Albach-Retty.*

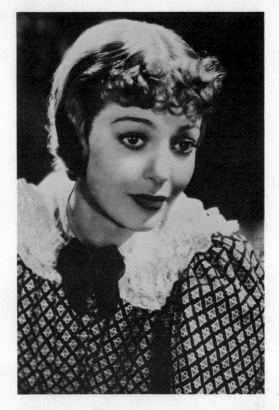

236

This beautiful American leading lady began her screen career at the age of 15. She won an Oscar for her role in *The Farmer's Daughter*. She had her own TV show for seven years.

1. *Gretchen Young.*   2. *Loretta McLoughlin.*
3. *Lori Youngstein.*

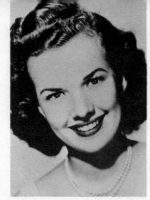

237

This petite, vivacious American actress made many Hollywood films in the forties. She made it big with her TV series called *The Gale Storm Show* and *My Little Margie.*

1. *Josephine Cottle.*   2. *Gale Sturmm.*
3. *Bobbi Anderson.*

238

She made few talkies, but was a great favorite in silent films and made several Hollywood films during the forties.

1. *Evelyn Bent.*   2. *Eve Bretwood.*
3. *Mary Elizabeth Riggs.*

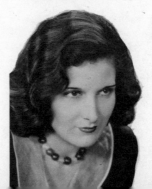

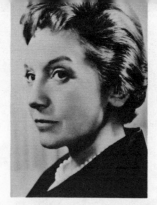

239

A German leading lady who settled in Britain in the thirties. She was brilliant in *Catherine the Great.*

1. *Elizabeth Ettel.*   2. *Elizabeth Wayne.*
3. *Liz Brechen.*

240

She went directly from college to Hollywood and scored heavily as a leading lady. She appeared on TV in *Mr. and Mrs. North* and *My Favorite Martian.*

1. *Clara Busch.*   2. *Barbara B. Czukor.*
3. *Babe Britain.*

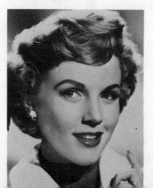

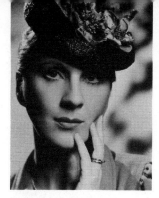

241

This fine English stage actress scored heavily as the heroine of *Cavalcade* in the early thirties.

1. *Dorothy Cox.*   2. *Diane Winnard.*
3. *Dina Wineapple.*

242

She played child parts in the mid-twenties and became a leading lady in American films, usually in gentle roles.

1. *Anita L. Fremault.*   2. *Anita Apple.*
3. *Anne Lawton.*

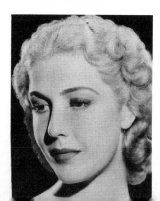

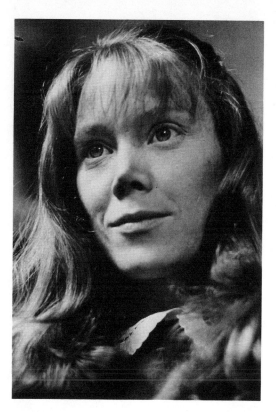

243

A fine actress who "scared" millions in her role in *Carrie* and won an Oscar for *Coal Miner's Daughter.*

1. *Sally Anne Sparton.*
2. *Carrie "Sis" Carlton.*
3. *Mary Elizabeth Spacek.*

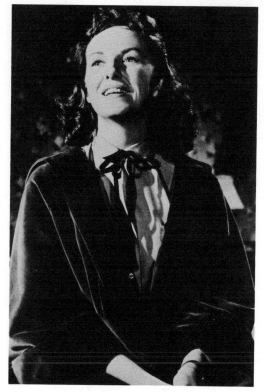

244

This American actress usually plays roles of shy or nervous women. She was memorable in *Another Part of the Forest.*

1. *Elizabeth Boger.*
2. *Betsy Loger.*
3. *Betty Moder.*

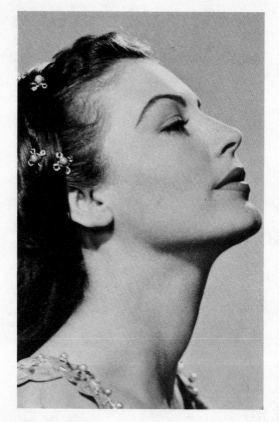

245

An American beauty and leading lady of the forties and fifties who was once voted one of the world's most beautiful women.

1. *Lucy Johnson.*   2. *Sarah Dineen.*
3. *Jane Pauley.*

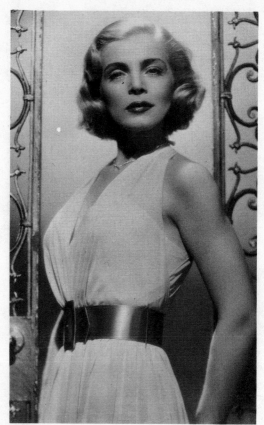

246

A sultry American leading lady of the forties who had a distinctive husky voice.

1. *Elizabeth Scotfield.*   2. *Emma Matzo.*
3. *Liz Walker.*

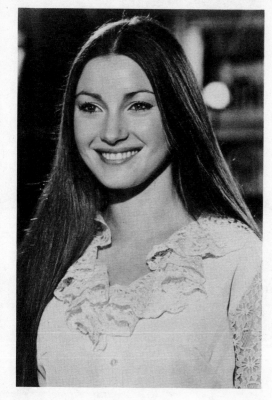

247

This talented British actress starred as a depraved female in John Steinbeck's epic *East of Eden* on TV.

1. *Joyce Penelope Frankenburg.*
2. *Debbie Brown.*
3. *Bonita Granville Wrather*

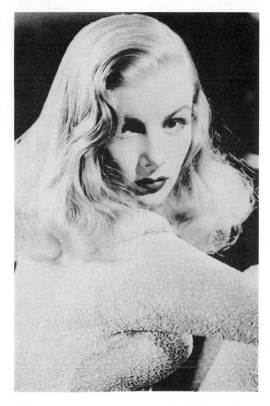

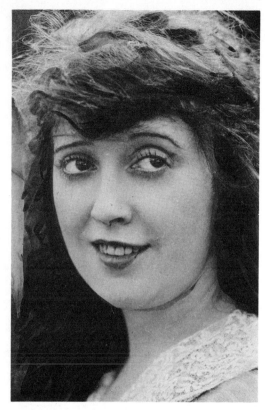

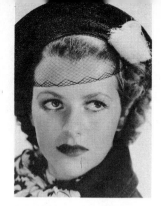

250

She was a special adviser on consumer affairs to President Johnson and was a great favorite of TV viewers and stage-goers.

1. *Betty Choate.*   2. *Elizabeth France.*
3. *Beth Winship.*

251

A prominent TV personality who graced the small screen for many years, especially as a panelist on game shows. She also appeared in many films.

1. *Eileen Stavis.*   2. *Arline Kazanjian.*
3. *Arlene Judgemento.*

248

She was a petite leading lady whose "peek-a-boo bang" (long blond hair obscuring one eye) became an American craze in the early forties.

1. *Vera Lakefish.*
2. *Constance Ockleman.*
3. *Kim Stahl.*

249

She was a great star of silent movies and an equally facile comedienne.

1. *Norma Mabelline.*
2. *Mabel Fortescue.*
3. *Mabel Fullerton.*

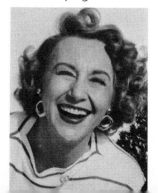

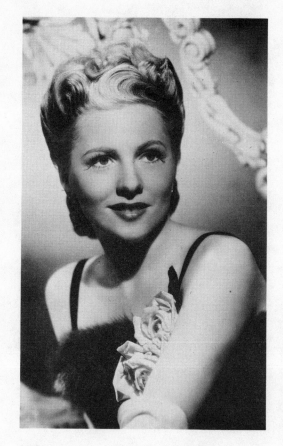

252

An American actress born in Japan. She has a sister who is also an Academy Award actress.

1. *Joan de Havilland.*   2. *Joanne Fountain.*
3. *Joan d'Arc-Fontayne.*

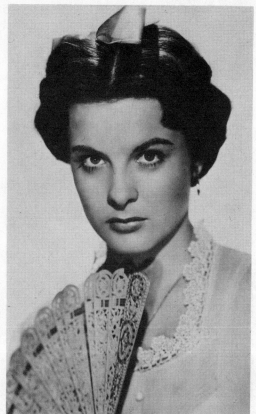

253

An attractive American leading lady who retired to marry millionaire recluse Howard Hughes.

1. *Jeanette Peterson.*   2. *Jean Pietro.*
3. *Elizabeth J. Peters.*

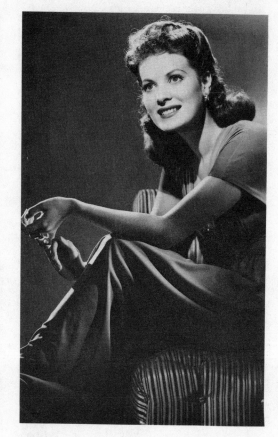

254

A striking red-haired Irish leading lady who became a big star in American films.

1. *Mary O'Hare.*   2. *Maureen Fitzsimmons.*
3. *Maureen O'Toole.*

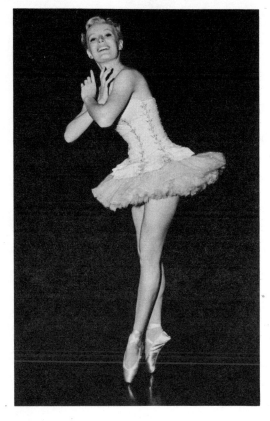

255

She achieved stardom in the role of the late dancer Marilyn Miller. She is married to actor Fred MacMurray.

1. *June Stovenour.*   2. *June Stopover.*
3. *June August.*

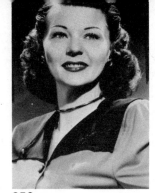

256

She was married to Ozzie Nelson, bandleader of radio fame, for many years. She was a leading lady in American films and romantic comedies and musicals in the thirties, and appeared with Ozzie on TV for ten years in *Ozzie and Harriet.*

1. *Harriette Hills.*   2. *Harriet Hilltop.*
3. *Peggy Lou Snyder.*

257

Once called the "most photographed model in the world," she became a leading lady in American films.

1. *Mara Inhaste.*   2. *Marilyn Watts.*
3. *Mary Cordrey.*

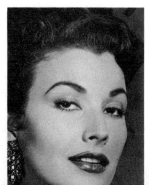

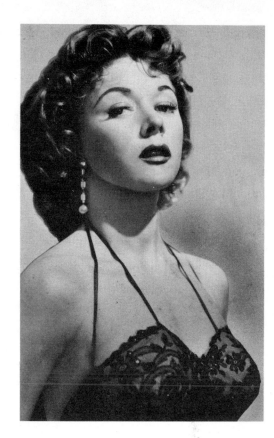

258

A sexy American actress who portrayed offbeat roles as a sultry blonde. She won an Academy Award for her role in *The Bad and the Beautiful.*

1. *Gloria Hallward.*   2. *Gloria Grahm.*
3. *Gloria Graham-Bell.*

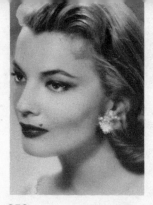

259

Another beautiful American actress who played leading romantic roles opposite many stars in the forties.

1. *Sherman Poole.*   2. *Virginia Beech.*
3. *Gilberta Virgin.*

260

She usually played smart women roles and was a leading lady in American films in Hollywood. She also produced successful TV shows, notably the *Perry Mason* series.

1. *Margaret Fitzpatrick.*
2. *Gail McCormick.*   3. *Patricia Gale.*

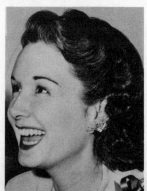

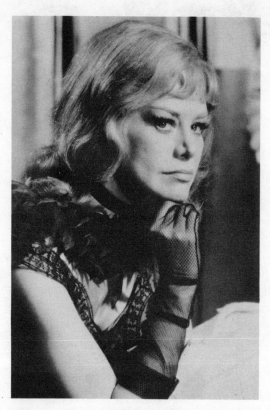

261

A former artist and film cartoonist, she appeared on the German stage, then in films. She came to Hollywood and wrote a best-seller, *The Gift Horse.*

1. *Marlise Pieratt.*   2. *Hilda Kopf.*
3. *Hildegarde Knef.*

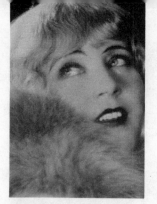

262

A great heart-throb on the silent screen, she was a former dancer who appeared in flashy movie roles.

1. *Mae Westland.*
2. *Marie Adrienne Koenig.*   3. *May Mirror.*

263

This luscious Polish-Austrian leading lady made some international films and then settled in Hollywood to make films in the thirties and forties.

1. *Natalie Bierle.*   2. *Tala Burrell.*
3. *Tallulah Birel.*

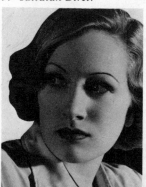

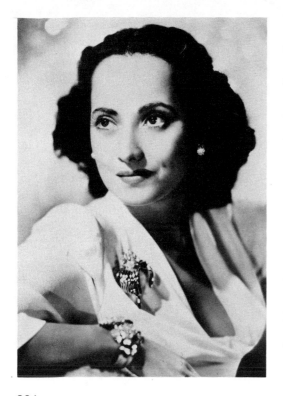

264

This lovely British leading lady was educated in India and came to Hollywood via Britain, where she was discovered working as a dance hostess. She captivated American audiences as Anne Boleyn in *The Private Life of Henry VIII*.

1. *Estelle O. M. Thompson.*
2. *Merle O'Brien.*   3. *Myrtle Beronne.*

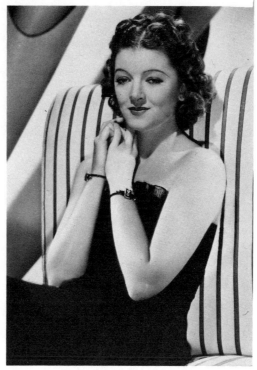

265

She is probably best remembered as "Nora Charles," the wife of "Nick Charles," ably played by William Powell in *The Thin Man*. She is still considered a big star.

1. *Myrna Williams.*
2. *Myrna Boysenberry.*
3. *Myrna Woodloy.*

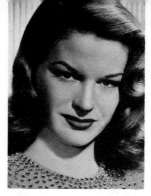

266

A very talented American actress, daughter of a famous Hollywood director-producer, she was born in Hollywood, California.

1. *Katie Stephens.*   2. *Gloria Wood.*
3. *Katherine Steeves.*

267

An American actress who was born in Portland, Oregon. She started in vaudeville and then moved on to musical comedy and films.

1. *Ona Wolcott.*   2. *Ona Cox.*
3. *Ona Monster.*

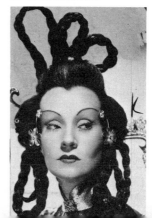

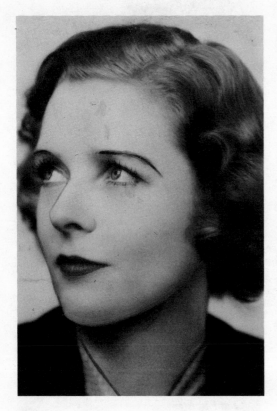

268

An American actress, born in 1895, who became one of the silent screen's best-known actresses. She later appeared on the stage in a featured role in *There's Always a Breeze*.

1. *Daphne Wayne.*   2. *Blanche Resier.*
3. *Ethel Moore.*

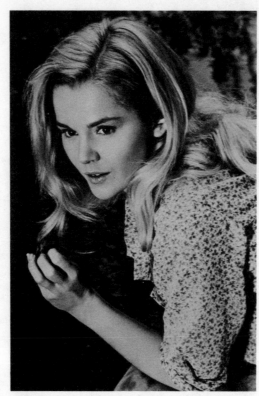

269

A fine American actress, born in 1943, who has appeared in scores of films. She is also an accomplished TV actress who is seen frequently on the small screen.

1. *Susan Ker Weld.*   2. *Tuesday Wilde.*
3. *Toots Wellde.*

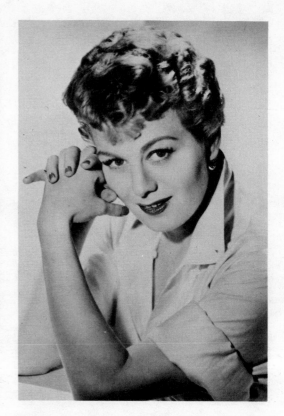

270

A talented American leading lady and character actress nominated many times for Best Actress by the Academy of Motion Picture Arts and Sciences.

1. *Shirley Schrift.*   2. *Shirley Shelle.*
3. *Sara Jane Winter.*

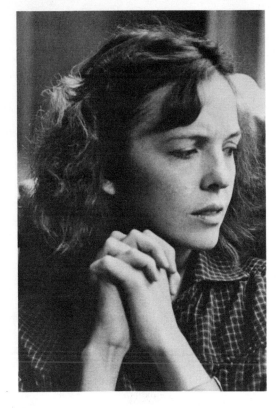

271

A very talented young actress who appears in many films by Woody Allen. She was excellent in *Looking for Mr. Goodbar* and in more recent films like *Annie Hall*.

1. *Deedee Baker.*　2. *Diane Hall.*
3. *Diana Keefer.*

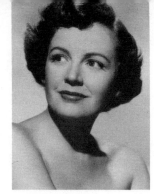

272

A former child actress, this British-born beauty came to Hollywood where she usually played "good" girls. She appeared on TV in *Kate*.

1. *Phyllis Pickerel.*　2. *Phyllis Bickle.*
3. *Phyllis Convert.*

273

She began as a model and developed into a fine American actress as well as TV star. She was married to the late Bobby Darin, the singer-actor.

1. *Alexandra Zuck.*　2. *Sandra Sands.*
3. *Sandra Diesel.*

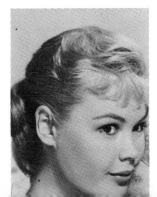

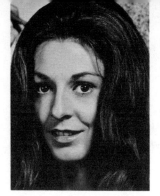

274

This talented actress appeared in many films with great success, as well as in several TV shows that received rave notices.

1. *Jane Quigley.*　2. *Jean Potter.*
3. *Alexandra Jayne Burke.*

275

This beautiful Italian actress made a big hit in the British film *The Third Man* in the late forties.

1. *Rue de Vallee.*　2. *Valerie Valdez.*
3. *Alida Maria Altenburger.*

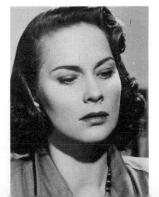

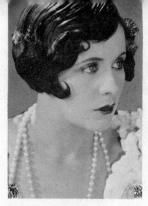

276

Not to be confused with the actress above, she was an American leading lady in silent films who retired to marry actor Charles Farrell.

1. *Virginia Colorado.*
2. *Virginia McSweeney.*   3. *Virginia Vallely.*

277

This demure, pretty American actress was a leading lady in silent movies during the twenties.

1. *Augusta Apple.*   2. *Lily Lee.*
3. *Leila Leeward.*

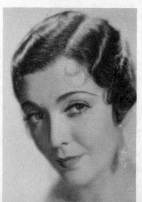

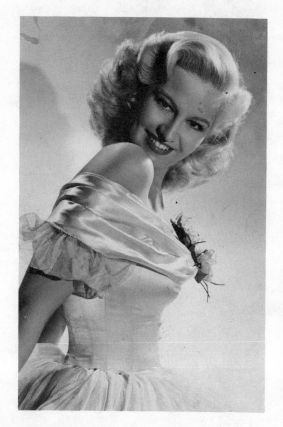

278

This beautiful, blond American actress played in many B-pictures in the forties through the sixties, and in a TV series, *Bus Stop 61.*

1. *Mary Crosby.*   2. *Maxwell Carr.*
3. *Marvel Maxwell.*

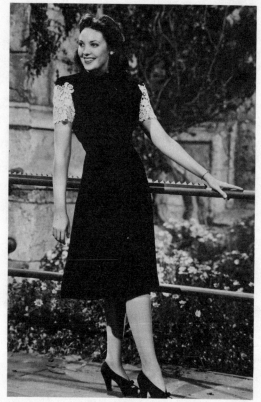

279

This wide-eyed American leading lady of the forties appeared in scores of movies, notably *It Happened Tomorrow.*

1. *Linda Darwell.*   2. *Lena Darnell.*
3. *Manetta Eloisa Darnell.*

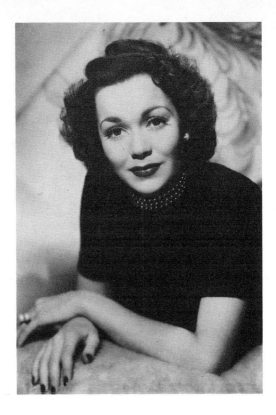

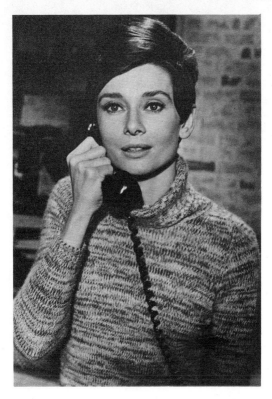

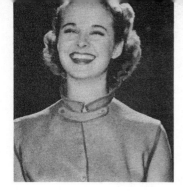

282

This beautiful actress became a leading lady in American films and was at her peak as a troublesome teenager in the forties.

1. *Mona Lisa Cottle.* 2. *Monica Freeman.*
3. *Mona Foreman.*

283

This pretty American actress was once married to William Holden. She appeared in scores of films as an ingenue before she graduated to more mature roles.

1. *Brenda Huston.* 2. *Ardis Ankerson.*
3. *Brenda Martin-Boynton.*

280

An Academy Award winner for her sterling portrayal of a mute in Johnny Belinda and a great character actress, she appeared on TV in *Falcon Crest*.

1. *Sarah Jane Fulks.* 2. *Joanne Belinda.*
3. *Jane Wiman-Strotter.*

281

This Belgium-born actress of Dutch-Irish parentage rose rapidly to stardom in American films after small roles in British films.

1. *Audrey Hepburn-Ruston.*
2. *Audrey Hepburn-Rills.*
3. *Audrey Hepburn-Bern.*

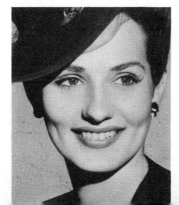

95

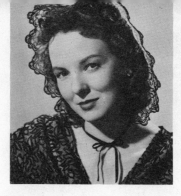

284

This British actress, in the U.S.A. since the late thirties, was a regular panelist of TV's *It's News to Me*.

1. *Joanna Winnifrith.*
2. *Anna Leighton-Jones.*   3. *Ann Boylene.*

285

An American film actress and comedienne who appeared as a Brooklynese character actress in innumerable films.

1. *Jean Verhagen.*   2. *Jean Metabolis.*
3. *Jeanne Cosmos.*

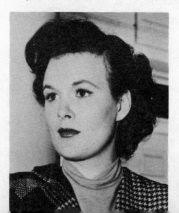

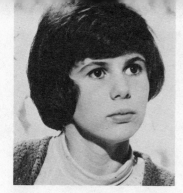

286

This talented actress made a big hit opposite John Wayne in *True Grit*.

1. *Kim Taylor.*   2. *Zerby Denby.*
3. *Darlene Kirby.*

287

She's a great French-American stage and screen star with experience on the New York stage.

1. *Andrea Roi.*   2. *Andrea Kingsbuty.*
3. *Georgetta Barry.*

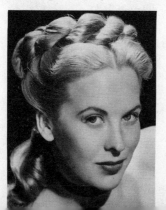

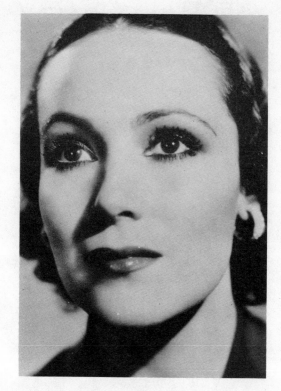

288

This beautiful Mexican actress was a cousin to silent movie actor Roman Novarro. She had her portrait painted by the famous artist Diego Rivera.

1. *Dorothy del Rio.*
2. *Lolita Dolores Martinez.*
3. *Dolores Martinez Asunsolo.*

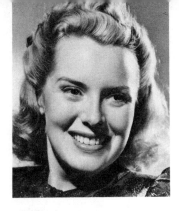

289

This American leading lady was a photographer's model and fashion model. She appeared in many films during the forties and fifties.

1. *Brenda Lynch.*   2. *Betty Leabo.*
3. *Brenda Jordon.*

290

A beautiful leading lady in American films who married screenwriter Arthur Sheekman, known for his Marx Brothers scripts.

1. *Gloria S. Finch.*   2. *Gloria Barron.*
3. *Gladys Steward.*

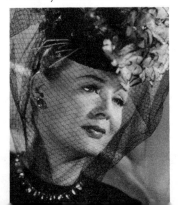

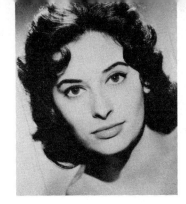

291

This fine actress is an American leading lady who has great stage experience.

1. *Ina Berg.*   2. *Ina Rosenberg.*
3. *Ina Begin.*

292

This beauty began her career in American films as a child star and graduated to leading lady roles.

1. *Dawn Paris.*   2. *Shirley Anton.*
3. *Anna Short.*

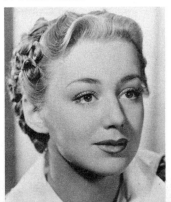

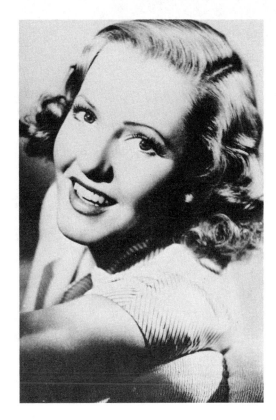

293

This cute, squeaky-voiced American leading lady, popular in the thirties and forties, specialized in social comedy; she made many Hollywood films.

1. *Gladys Greene.*   2. *Jeanette Parkson.*
3. *Jean Parks-Talston.*

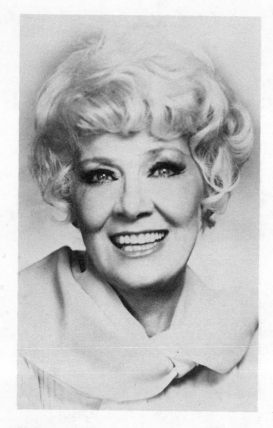

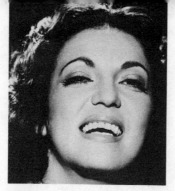

295

She is a spirited Mexican actress who has made many hit Hollywood films. She appears on TV in character roles.

1. *Katie Liebowitz.*
2. *Maria Christina J. Garcia.*
3. *Kathryn Cantinflas.*

296

She was a temperamental Mexican leading lady of the thirties, best remembered with Leon Errol in the *Mexican Spitfire* series.

1. *Maria y Valloz.*
2. *Maria Guadaloupe Villalobos.*
3. *Valerie Acapulco.*

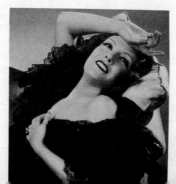

294

This blond American leading lady, formerly in vaudeville, played "Blondie," the comic strip heroine, in two films a year for ten years.

1. *Carol Ellis.*   2. *Carol Curley.*
3. *Dorothy McNulty.*

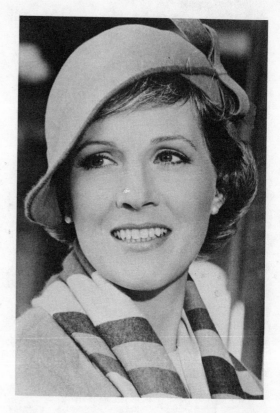

297

This lovely British actress is best known for her Oscar-winning role in *Mary Poppins*, as well as *The Sound of Music* and many other American films.

1. *Julia Wells.*   2. *Julie Neal.*
3. *Judy Wellington.*

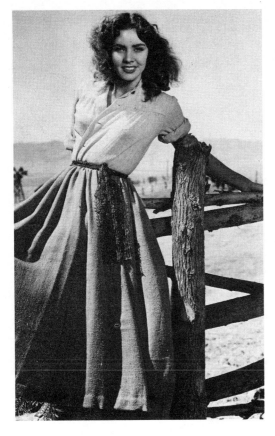

298

This beautiful and multitalented actress won an Oscar for her role in *The Song of Bernadette*.

1. *Phyllis Ainsley.*   2. *Phyllis Isley.*
3. *Jenny Johnson.*

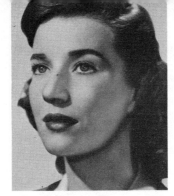

299

This pretty Canadian leading lady had a brief Hollywood career in the late forties before settling in England.

1. *Lois Max.*   2. *Lois Martin.*
3. *Lois Hooker.*

300

A beautiful actress who began in films about the same time as Doris Day. She is a well-known American leading lady who began with operatic training. She is also seen frequently on TV.

1. *Donna Mae Jaden.*   2. *Janice Pagler.*
3. *Jane Rossiter.*

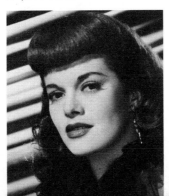

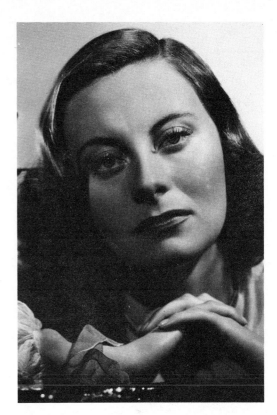

301

This beautiful French actress was a leading lady from the mid-thirties. She captivated American audiences too, especially in *La Symphonie Pastorale*.

1. *Simone Roussel.*   2. *Preal Weinstein.*
3. *Annie Gaybis.*

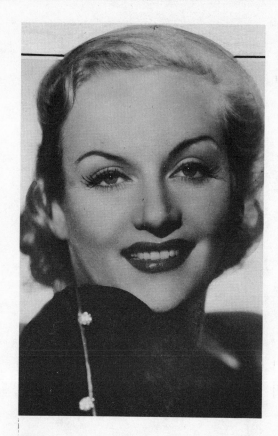

302

This beautiful blond comedienne was an American leading lady of the thirties. She was married to Clark Gable.

1. *Judy Parsons.*　2. *Jane Alice Peters.*
3. *Carol Lazarlus.*

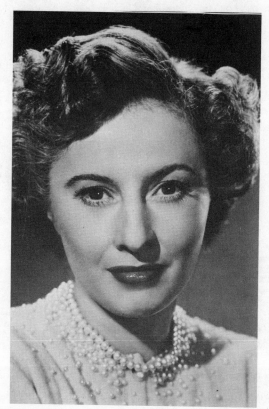

303

A major American movie star whose memorable performance in *Double Indemnity* is hailed as a classic. She made it big in TV in *The Big Valley*.

1. *Ruby Stevens.*　2. *Barbara Stanton.*
3. *Bebe Stratton.*

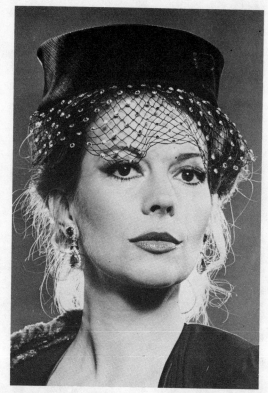

304

She was a child star who became a dramatic film actress later in life. She is best remembered for *Marjorie Morningstar* and *West Side Story*. She was married to Robert Wagner.

1. *Natasha Gurdin.*　2. *Susan Brady.*
3. *Natlie Woodley.*

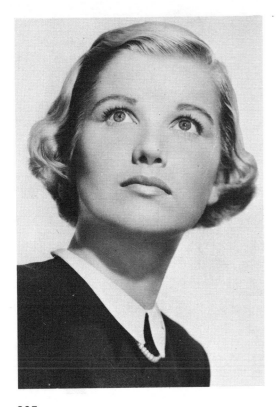

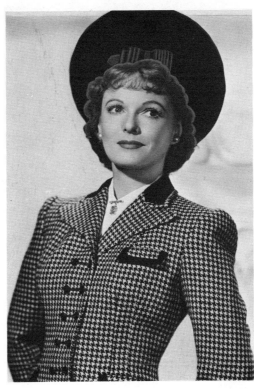

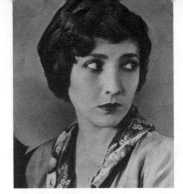

307

This is a rare photograph of a vivacious, petite leading lady in Hollywood films in the early twenties. She was in films since childhood and occasionally played cameo roles.

1. *Bethel Amour.*   2. *Bess Lovelace.*
3. *Juanita Horton.*

308

Known throughout America as "The Queen of Shimmy," this Polish-born dancer made films in Hollywood in the early thirties.

1. *Elyse Goldberg.*
2. *Marianna Michalska.*
3. *Barbara J. Parsons.*

305

She is best known on TV as J.R.'s mother in *Dallas*. In films she usually played nice, placid girls, opposite some of the screen's biggest stars.

1. *Barbara Streisser.*
2. *Barbara G. Lewis.*
3. *Babs Procter.*

306

This British actress was a former chorus dancer who built up a formidable film gallery of historical heroines. She was also a fine stage actress and producer.

1. *Anne Burjou.*   2. *Arlene Nagle.*
3. *Marjorie Robertson.*

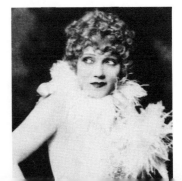

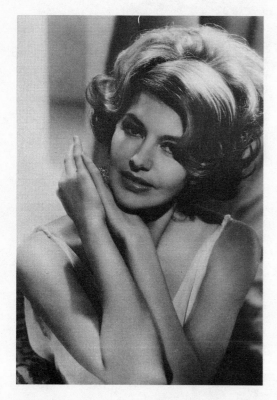

309

This beautiful dancer is married to Tony Martin. A long-legged, stylish American actress, she was the leading lady in many MGM musicals.

1. *Charlotte Cerise*.
2. *Carlotta Cherrystone*.
3. *Tula Ellice Finklea*.

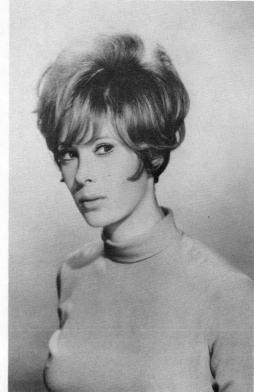

310

This statuesque actress appears frequently on TV and is an excellent comedienne. She has made several good films.

1. *Kate Williamson*.   2. *Edy Williams*.
3. *Jill Oppenheim*.

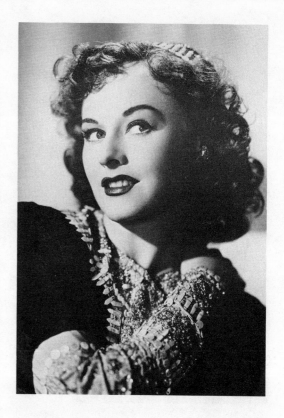

311

A bright and witty leading lady of the forties, who started as a Goldwyn Girl and advanced to starring roles with Charlie Chaplin, whom she later married.

1. *Paulette Francoise*.   2. *Marion Levy*.
3. *Madelaine Gardot*.

6. FUNNY PEOPLE

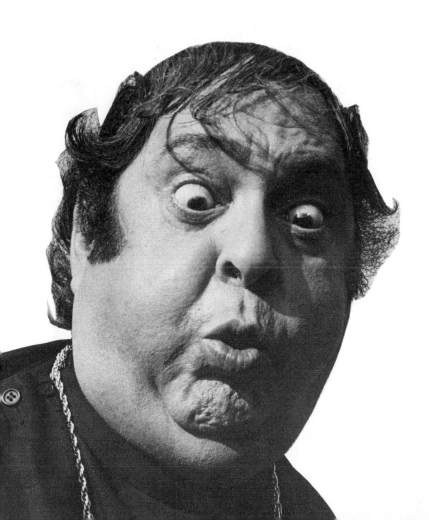

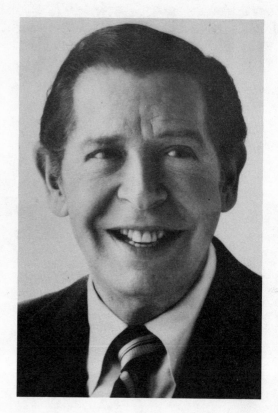

312

Here is "Mr. Television" himself. He is one of America's most able comedians and has captivated audiences on stage, screen, TV, and in clubs.

1. *Harvey Chertok.* 2. *Maurice Lazarus.*
3. *Milton Berlinger.*

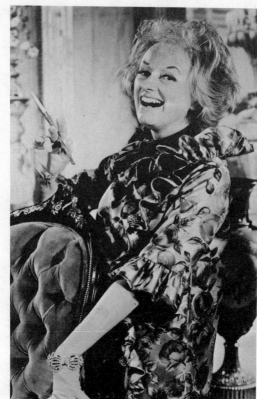

313

This remarkable comedienne began as a zany, brash actress. She appears on television and is a favorite with club-goers.

1. *Ada Phyllis Driver.* 2. *Judy Parsons.*
3. *Linda Gutstein.*

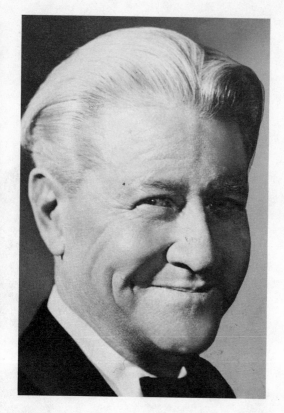

314

This cheerful American comic actor, who was best known for his startled "double take," began in vaudeville. He made his film debut in 1927 in *Finders Keepers* and continued for years.

1. *Lewis D. Offield.* 2. *Kenneth Gore.*
3. *Bob Weaver.*

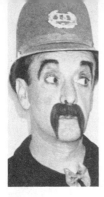

315

This Australian comedian came to America and made silent films in Hollywood, most of them of the slapstick variety.

1. *Edward C. Parkhurst.*   2. *Harold Fraser.*
3. *Jack Thomas.*

316

This diminutive, dapper English comedian was a master of the pratfall on stage. He came from a famous family of clowns. He made two-reel silent comedies that are considered masterpieces.

1. *Lance Landersino.*
2. *Henry George Lupino.*   3. *Fred Langone.*

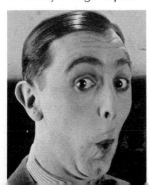

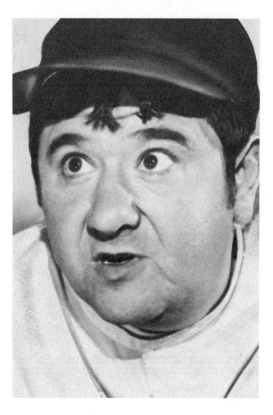

317

This tubby, fast-talking story-teller is among the most versatile comedians in America. He appears frequently in nightclubs and occasionally on TV. He also made a TV series, *Stanley.*

1. *Leonard Hacker.*   2. *Sam Heilner.*
3. *Isaac Fisher.*

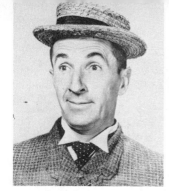

318

A very funny visual comedian who rose from the ranks of vaudeville to musical comedies, films, and TV.

1. *Benjamin Bluestein.*
2. *Benjamin Bernstein.*   3. *David Blue.*

319

The co-star of the popular TV series *Doc*, she has appeared in many successful movies and stage productions. She started out with Henry Fonda, Margaret Sullavan, and Gertrude Lawrence.

1. *Mary Wickenhauser.*   2. *Mary Rosen.*
3. *Marcy Sandler.*

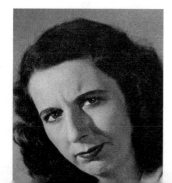

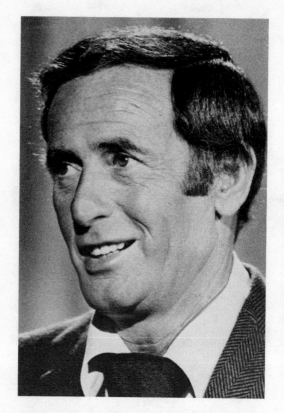

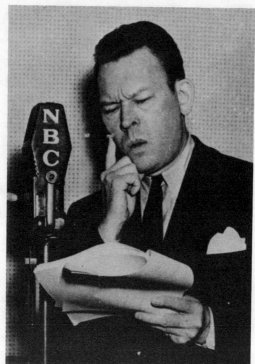

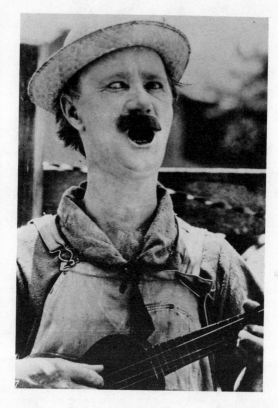

320

A great standup comedian who made it big on TV as a humorist and master of ad libs. He is known for his successful TV series and several zany American films.

1. *Brett Paul.*   2. *Joseph Gottlieb.*
3. *Sid Grossman.*

321

This baggy-eyed humorist spoke with a nasal twang which endeared him to millions of radio fans during the thirties and forties. He made several Hollywood films and "feuded" with Jack Benny on radio and TV.

1. *Jim Sullivan.*   2. *Paul Sullivan.*
3. *John Florence Sullivan.*

322

This cross-eyed comedian was a popular actor in short, slapstick silent comedies in the twenties. He was a vaudevillian before becoming a Hollywood actor.

1. *Bob Perlstein.*   2. *Bernard Turpin.*
3. *Ben Cohen.*

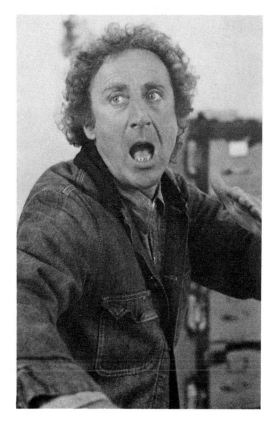

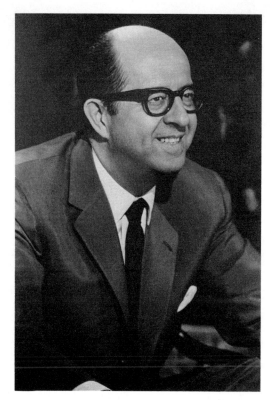

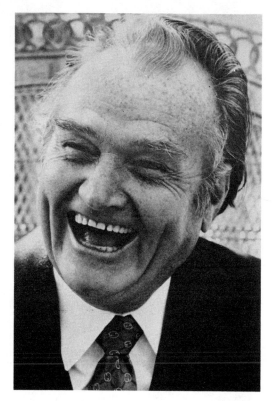

323

He's a very funny actor who appears frequently in films produced by Mel Brooks. He's also an accomplished stage actor.

1. *Gerald Silberman.*   2. *William Canby.*
3. *Walter Hunt.*

324

This very funny man is a great musical comedy star and his own TV series, *You'll Never Get Rich*, made "Sgt. Bilko" a household word in America.

1. *Philip Silversmith.*   2. *Gene Shields.*
3. *Waldo Graham.*

325

One of the funniest comedians ever to grace the stage, screen, radio, and TV. He also made many Hollywood movies. On radio and TV he delighted millions weekly on his own show.

1. *Arthur Skelton.*   2. *Sheldon Skelton.*
3. *Richard Skelton.*

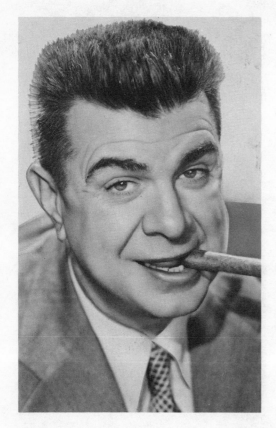

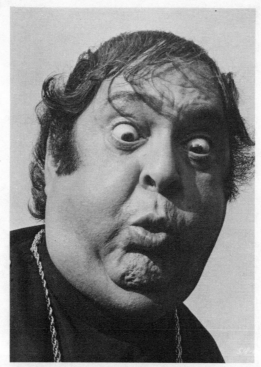

327

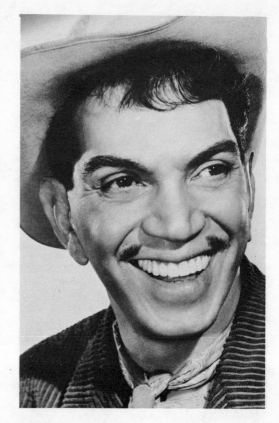

326

An American comic and entertainer who specializes in rare home-movie showings of celebrities.

1. *Fred Pierce.*   2. *Jack Stein.*
3. *Don Court.*

He was a great American character actor, starring in such modern classics as *Fiddler on the Roof* and *A Funny Thing Happened on the Way to the Forum.* He got his nickname from the low grades he got in school.

1. *Samuel Mostel.*   2. *Harry Mostel.*
3. *Robert Mostel.*

328

This Mexican clown, acrobat, and bullfighter came to the States and made notable films, such as *Pepe* and *Around the World in Eighty Days.*

1. *Al Krivin.*   2. *Julio Cesar.*
3. *Mario Moreno.*

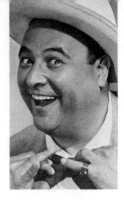

329

One of the original "insult" comedians, much in the vein of Don Rickles. He appeared in films and in nightclubs, where he had a great following.

1. *Bob Daly.*   2. *Thomas Jack.*
3. *Leonard Lebitsky.*

330

This fine comedian was a screen favorite, with lots of stage and TV experience. He appeared on TV in *Baretta* and his own series.

1. *S. Yewell Tompkins.*   2. *Dick Sinnot.*
3. *Thomas Yule, Sr.*

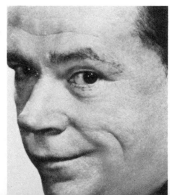

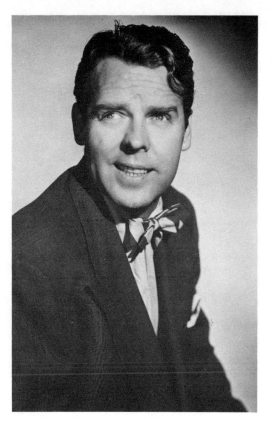

331

This actor is best remembered for his portrayal of "Dagwood Bumstead" in the *Blondie* series of 38 movies in 12 years.

1. *Lee Fields.*   2. *Arthur Silverlake.*
3. *Albert Kramer.*

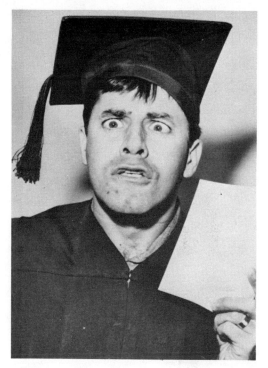

332

When he teamed with Dean Martin they became the most successful comedy team in America. He is also revered as a genius in Europe. He appears frequently on TV and in films, alone, having split with Martin in the fifties.

1. *Joseph Levitch.*   2. *Jeremiah Levitt.*
3. *Louis Jerrold.*

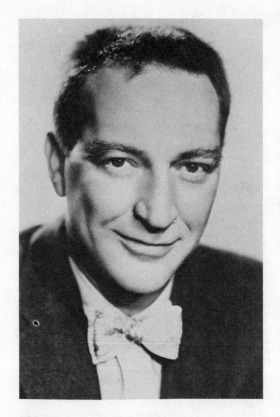

333

A very clever American comedian who was a big hit on radio and later on TV as host of *I've Got a Secret* and other programs, including his own show.

1. *Gerald Morrison.* 2. *Jerry More.*
3. *Thomas Morfit.*

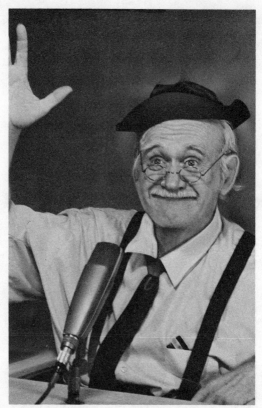

334

He was a favorite on TV's *Hollywood Squares* and appeared on *The Johnny Carson Show* frequently.

1. *Cliff Arquette.* 2. *Charles Mendelson.*
3. *Charles Whipple.*

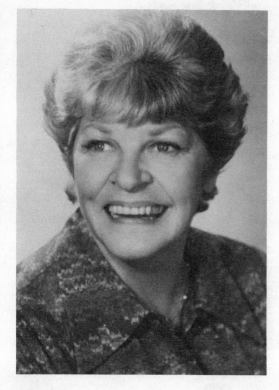

335

She's a wide-mouthed American comedienne and vocalist, popular on radio and TV as well as in many films. She had her own TV series, under her name, and also appeared in *The Bugaloos.*

1. *Martha Raymond.* 2. *Margaret O'Reed.*
3. *Martha Raytheon.*

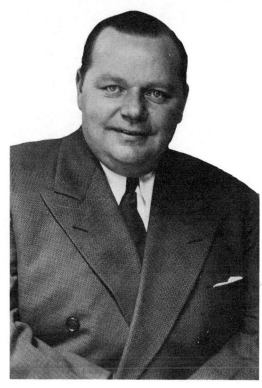

336

He was a grown-up fat boy of American silent cinema whose career was blemished by a 1921 scandal. Some of his silent two-reel films are still funny.

1. *Arthur Arbutus.*   2. *Arthur Buckley.*
3. *Roscoe Conklin Arbuckle.*

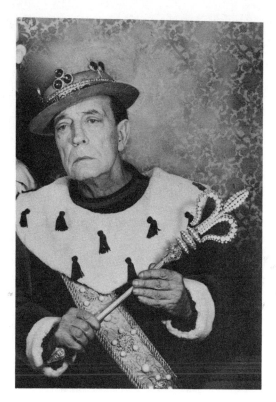

337

A great stone-faced comedian whose role in the film *The Navigator* was a masterpiece. He was nicknamed "Buster" by magician Harry Houdini.

1. *Joseph Francis Keaton, Jr.*
2. *Keith Roberts.*   3. *Keats van Egges.*

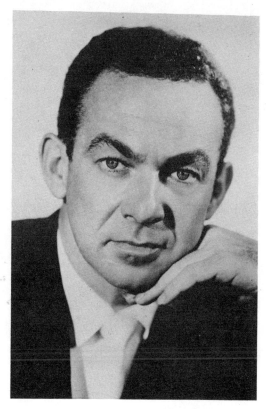

338

He is one of the brightest, most original comedians appearing on stage, TV, and in clubs and films. His brash style of humor is a delight.

1. *Jack Chakrin.*   2. *Truman Carroll.*
3. *Jack McMahon.*

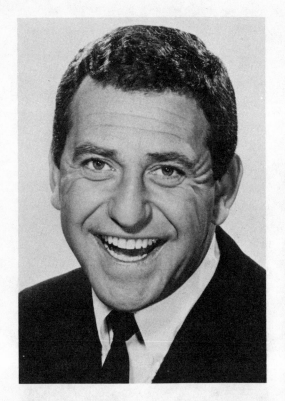

339

He is a very funny entertainer who was popular on children's TV shows. Our source reveals that he changed his name because it sounded too much like that of a soup and ketchup manufacturer's. (It's plausible!)

1. *Billy Campbell.* 2. *Milton Hines.*
3. *Henry Hormel.*

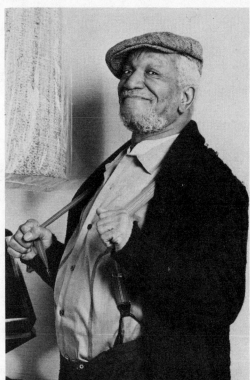

340

A talented actor who made stage appearances and recordings long before he was discovered by TV. He made a big hit with his series, *Sanford and Son.*

1. *John Elroy Sanford.* 2. *John Foxx.*
3. *Foxx Reddy.*

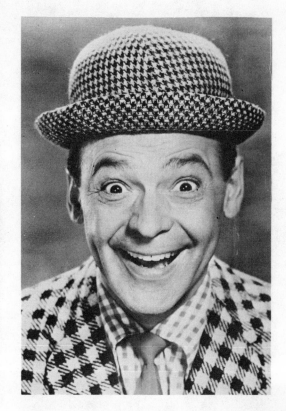

341

An American TV comedian who captivated children with his zany, simple humor. He starred in burleque, vaudeville, on the stage, and in films.

1. *Pincus Leff.* 2. *Lee Pinkerton.*
3. *Lee Pintner.*

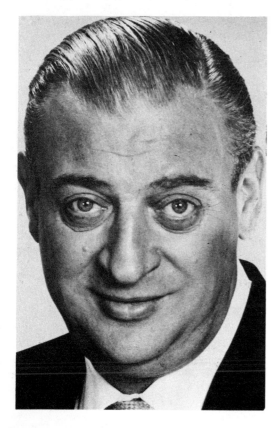

342

One of the funniest stand-up comics in the business today. He still "don't get no respect," but is respected by his peers as among the best.

1. *Jacob Cohen.*   2. *Rodney Fields.*
3. *Ronnie Danler.*

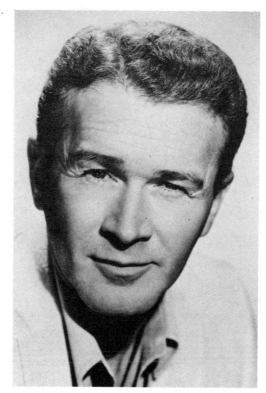

343

He is not only one of America's greatest comedians but won an Academy Award for his masterful role in *Sayonara*; yet, "No one gave me a dinner," he admits.

1. *Isaac Stern.*   2. *Aaron Chwatt.*
3. *Cyrus Evans.*

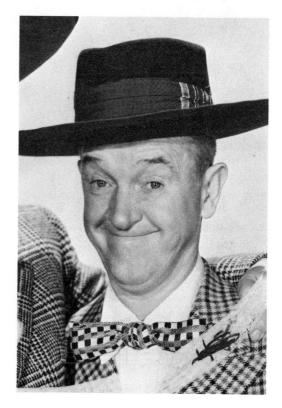

344

Half of a famous comedy team, he was a British-born comedian and won a special Academy Award in 1960. He was the butt of many of Hardy's (the fat one's) gags.

1. *Stan Lawrence.* 2. *Arthur Stanley Jefferson.*
3. *Morrie Roizman.*

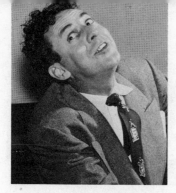

345

This fine American comic appeared in many one-reel films, notably the *Behind the Eight Ball* series. He also was a TV performer in the late forties.

1. *George Rice.* 2. *Leigh Montville.*
3. *Bob King.*

346

This wide-eyed, mustached screen comedian achieved fame in silent films and became a member of Mac Sennett's troupe. He also played bewildered policemen.

1. *Paul Tiberi.* 2. *Willian Veban.*
3. *William B. Harris.*

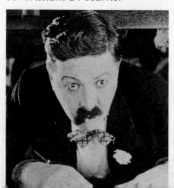

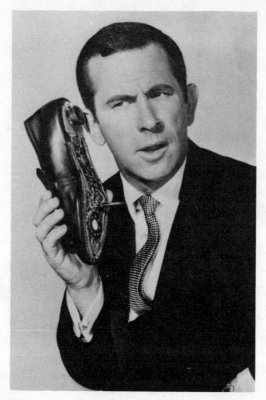

347

A very funny actor who starred in a smash TV show, *Get Smart*, playing the role of an "all-thumbs" secret agent who would make James Bond cry "U.N.C.L.E."

1. *Adam Donaldson.* 2. *Donald M. DeHart.*
3. *Donald Yarmy.*

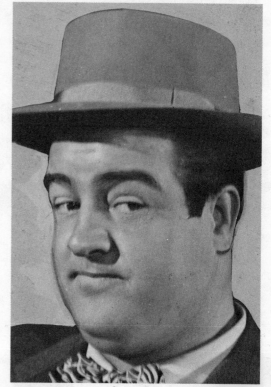

348

He was half of a famous comedy team. From burlesque they went into films and were favorites of millions. He was the dumpier and zanier of the two.

1. *Louis Untermeyer.* 2. *Louis Cristillo.*
3. *Hy Ciglio.*

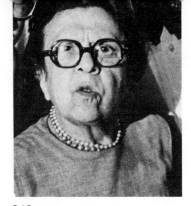

349

She was one of radio's funniest dialecticians and appeared as a regular with Fred Allen on the famous "Allen's Alley" segment of Fred's *Town Hall Tonight* coast-to-coast radio show.

1. *Ida Levin.*   2. *Minerva Pious.*
3. *Avis Savage.*

350

This American comedy actress achieved her greatest success on radio with Bob Hope. She also appeared in several films in the fifties.

1. *Barbara Jo Allen.*   2. *Vera McCarthy.*
3. *Henrietta Kissinger.*

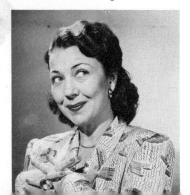

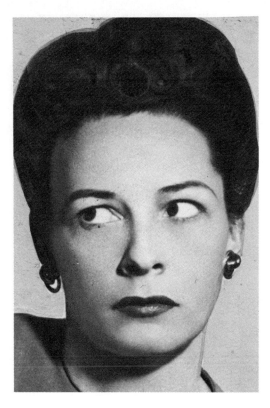

351

Here is an American comedienne who shouted songs, did acrobatic contortions, and was a feature in several light musicals of the forties. She also made many Hollywood movies.

1. *Catherine Dailey.*   2. *Karin Miller.*
3. *Gail Cassidy.*

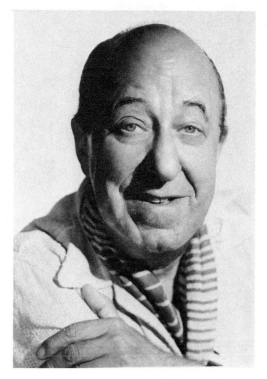

352

One of the nation's zaniest comedians, he was known on radio as "The Fire Chief." He was a great musical comedy entertainer and made several films in Hollywood. He has a son who is a talented actor.

1. *Isaiah Edwin Leopold.*   2. *Lester Smith.*
3. *Ed Peters.*

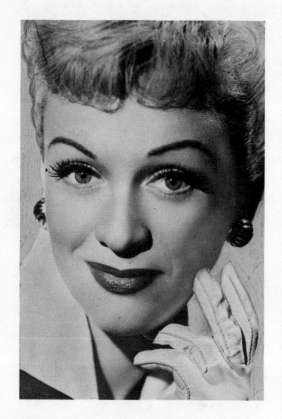

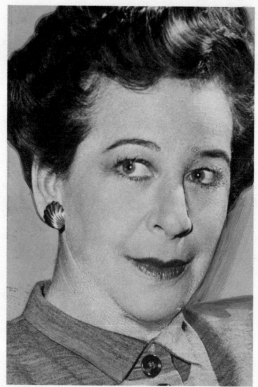

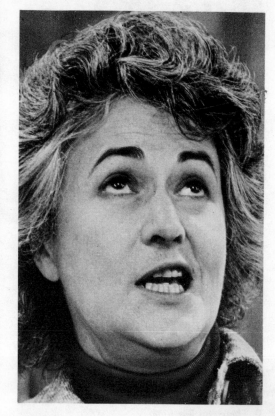

353

This tall, cool lady spent much of her screen career as a wise-cracking comedienne. Her TV and radio series, *Our Miss Brooks*, was a standout.

1. *Eunice Quedens.*   2. *Joan Franklin.*
3. *Joanne Montanus.*

354

She was one of America's leading comediennes in musical comedy. She scored heavily as "Baby Snooks" on radio, and her films, although infrequent, were memorable.

1. *Fanny Breistein.*   2. *Fanny Borach.*
3. *Fay Stein.*

355

She won a Tony for her stage role in *Mame*, and appears in films. Her TV series, *Maude*, was a huge success.

1. *Bernice Frankel.*   2. *Beatrice Arkin.*
3. *Bonnie Brooks.*

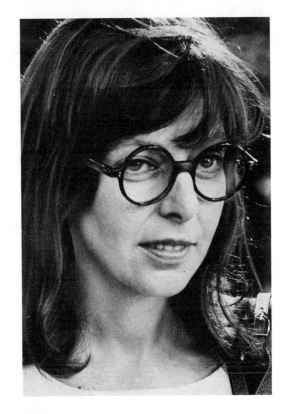

356

She is a brilliant comedienne who paired with Mike Nichols to create some of the zaniest situations ever heard. She is also a screenwriter and director.

1. *Eileen Prose.* 2. *Marcia Chmara.*
3. *Elaine Berlin.*

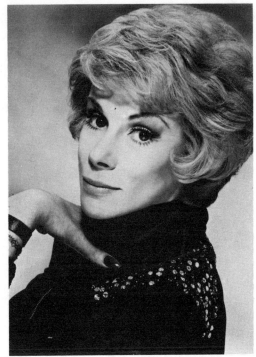

357

Many consider her to be the funniest comedienne in America. She is also a movie producer and appears frequently on *The Johnny Carson Show*. She may be seen in Las Vegas and other fashionable nightclub cities.

1. *Joan Molinsky.* 2. *Joan Riverdale.*
3. *Joan Smithers.*

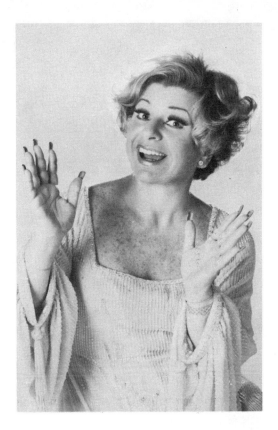

358

She was a popular nightclub and TV comedienne who was voted Comedienne of the Year in 1978 by the American Guild of Variety Artists.

1. *Totie Fieldston.* 2. *Toots Margolis.*
3. *Sophie Feldman.*

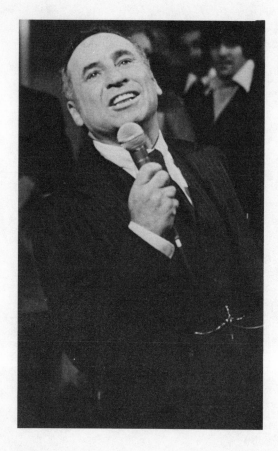

359

He's a producer, director, and actor in many of his zany films. He is married to Ann Bancroft.

1. *Melvyn Kaminsky.* 2. *Mel Simons.*
3. *Bernard Weinstock.*

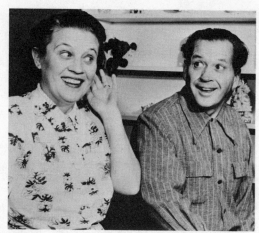

360

He was the male half of a famous radio comedy team. A feature of the program was weird sound effects, especially when he opened his closet door and the sound of its falling contents seemed to go on endlessly.

1. *Frank McGonagle.* 2. *Norm Crosby.*
3. *James Edward Jordan.*

361

She was the female half of the team and a perfect foil for her real-life husband. The program lasted over three decades and entertained millions.

1. *Paula Miller.* 2. *Marion Driscoll.*
3. *Yolanda Trigg.*

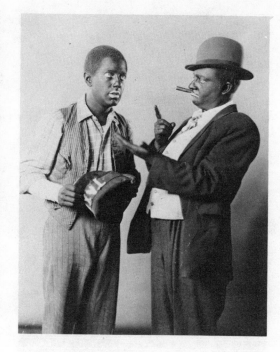

362

Two of the nation's most popular entertainers during the early days of radio. Whey they spoke—*everybody* listened!

Amos: 1. *Freeman F. Gosden.*
      2. *Joel Spiegel.*
      3. *Irving H. Ludwig.*
Andy: 1. *Card Walker.*
      2. *Charles Correll.*
      3. *Ken Behrens.*

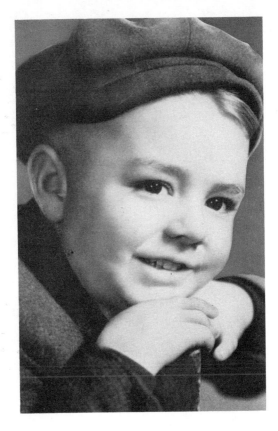

363

He was one of the best known kids in short comedies featuring the "Our Gang" kids. He was the "fat boy."

1. *David I. Stemerman.*   2. *Marty Ross.*
3. *George Emmett McFarland.*

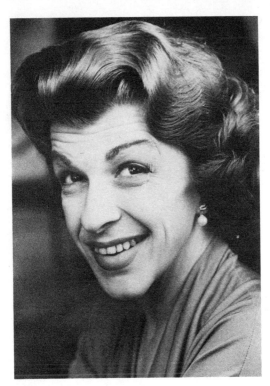

364

This brilliant comedienne has appeared on nearly every major TV show, after a brilliant stage career. She is best known as the mother in TV's *Rhoda*, and does a famous TV commercial for a paper-towel company.

1. *Anna Myrthle Swoyer.*   2. *Nancy Walters.*
3. *Nancy Baato.*

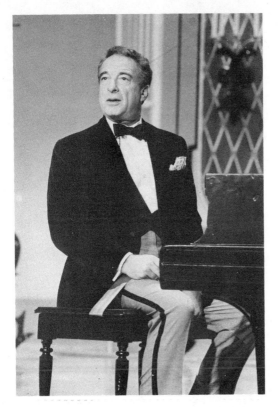

365

This Danish comedian and fine pianist has entertained millions of theatre-goers throughout the world. He has been cited by the Danish government.

1. *Victor Brodney.*   2. *Borge Rosenbaum.*
3. *George Borkman.*

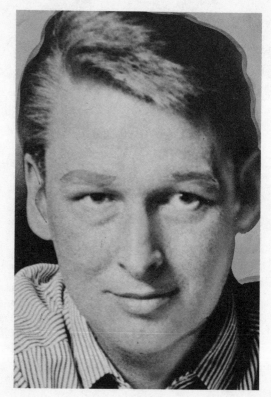

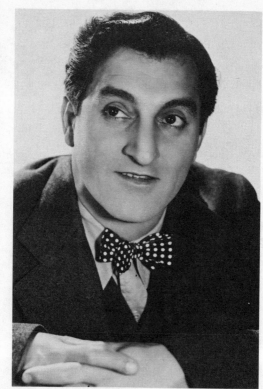

366

He made up a fine comedy team with Elaine May. He was a nightclub entertainer who became a successful stage and film director, winning an Oscar for *The Graduate*.

1. *Michael Steinberg.*   2. *Robert Luzzi.*
3. *Michael Peschkowsky.*

367

He began as a nightclub comedian and went on to make movies. He starred in *The Jazz Singer* and had his own TV show for seven lucrative years.

1. *Amos Jacobs.*   2. *Duane Dhlouly.*
3. *Daniel Thompson.*

7. CHARACTER PLAYERS

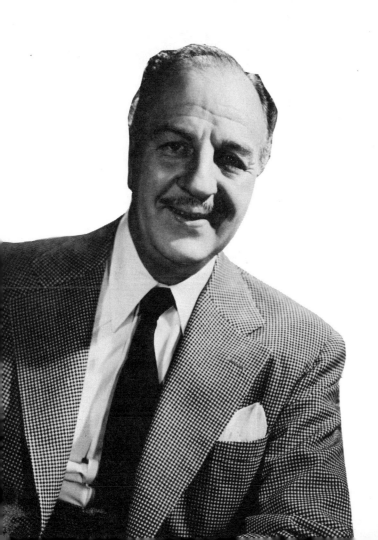

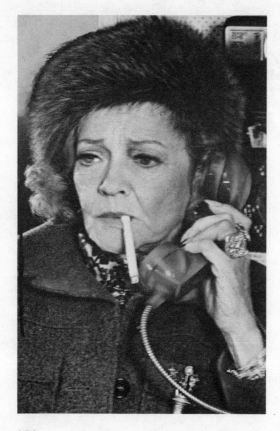

368

As a fragile, dark-eyed heroine in Hollywood films, she rose to stardom in strong character roles. She may be seen on TV frequently.

1. *Dawn Clayton.*   2. *Sophia Kosow.*
3. *Lois Armstrong.*

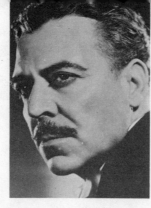

369

He is a humorous but often sinister Maltese character actor who came to Hollywood after an opera career and played many distinguished roles.

1. *Joseph Spurin-Calleja.*   2. *John Parks.*
3. *Michael Bogart.*

370

This great American character actor is a stage and screen/TV favorite.

1. *Harold Silverblatt.*   2. *Wynn Nathan.*
3. *Evan Dame.*

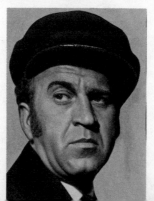

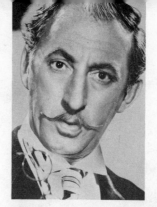

371

This great German actor made many successful American films and delighted millions with his comedy.

1. *Siegfried Aron.*   2. *Pierre Weis.*
3. *Chick Beesemyer*

372

This Canadian-born Norwegian character actor usually played amiably ineffectual foreign types. He had a delightful accent.

1. *Wasyl Matlaga.*   2. *John Oleson.*
3. *Tony De Mauro.*

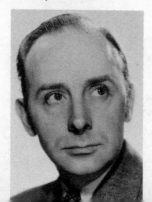

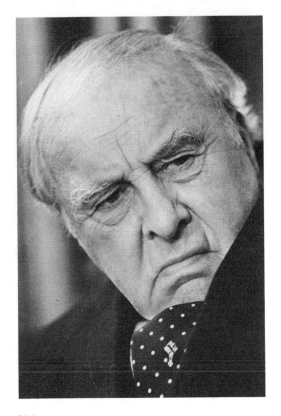

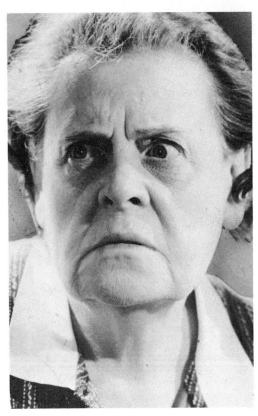

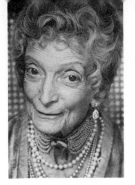

375

She was one of the oldest actresses actively appearing in films and on the stage. She was in her nineties and usually played eccentric roles.

1. *Dorothy Rosen.*   2. *Estelle Goodwin.*
3. *Edith Liebowitz.*

376

She was a brilliant character actress who was universally known as "Molly Goldberg" in the famous radio/TV series *The Goldbergs*. She had a TV series, *Mrs. G. Goes to College*, and appeared on the screen in *Molly*.

1. *Gertrude Edelstein.*   2. *Gertrude Bergholz.*
3. *Gertrude Berger.*

373

This fine character actor has become an actor-in-great-demand as a result of his immediate success as "The Professor" in *The Paper Chase*, both on TV and in the film.

1. *Len Ringquist.*   2. *John Mason.*
3. *Jacques Haussman.*

374

"The grand old lady of films," who made movies with Wallace Beery, notably *Tugboat Annie* at MGM.

1. *Leila Von Koerber.*   2. *Mary Saddler.*
3. *Margaret Whiting.*

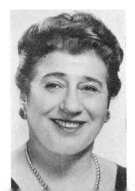

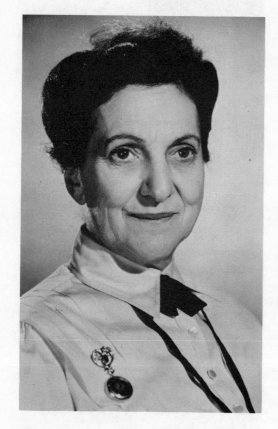

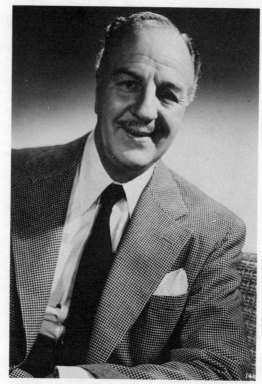

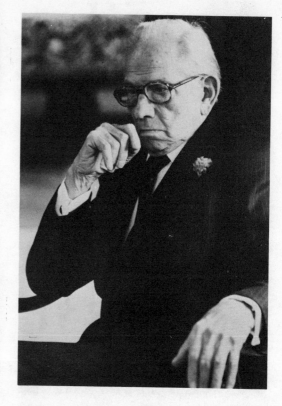

377

She was a distinguished actress who from early middle age played cantankerous or kindly old ladies in Hollywood films.

1. *Beulah Bondy.* 2. *Bella Bondage.*
3. *Bonnie Boolah.*

378

A great character actor whose roles on Broadway and Hollywood were unequalled in excellence.

1. *Anthony DeMauro.*
2. *Carl Henry Vogt.*
3. *Herbert Schmertz.*

379

This fine character actor won an Oscar for his role in *Hud*. He was a suave and polished leading man in many successful Hollywood films.

1. *Ron Miller.* 2. *Bill Moses.*
3. *Melvyn Hesselberg.*

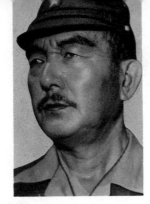

380

A fine Japanese actor and a popular star in silent films, he captivated American moviegoers with his role in *The Bridge on the River Kwai*.

1. *S. I. Hayakawa.*   2. *Eng-Hwi Kwa.*
3. *Kintaro Hayakawa.*

381

This gangly, slow-speaking, lethargic-like American black comedian was most popular during the thirties, when he appeared in many films.

1. *B. J. Fetchin.*   2. *Stephan Fechann.*
3. *Lincoln Perry.*

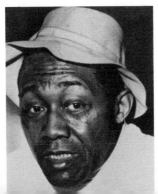

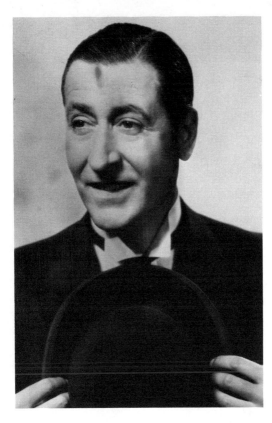

382

He portrayed the archetypical British butler on stage, screen, and TV. He is best known as Merv Griffin's sidekick on TV.

1. *Arthur Katz.*   2. *Arthur T. Veary.*
3. *Arthur Kronk.*

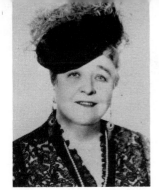

383

One of the great ladies of the cinema who won the Academy Award for her Best Supporting Actress role in *The Grapes of Wrath*.

1. *Patti Woodward.*   2. *Jane Darling.*
3. *Janice Sterling.*

384

She is a versatile American actress who made several films in Hollywood. Her greatest achievement was in TV's *Gunsmoke*, which ran for several years.

1. *Amanda Bleake.*   2. *Beverly Neill.*
3. *Besse Armadon.*

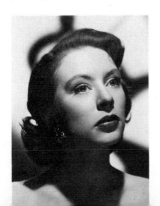

125

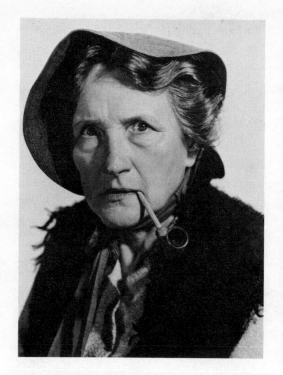

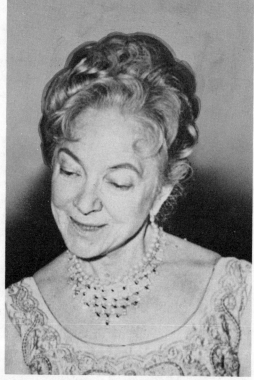

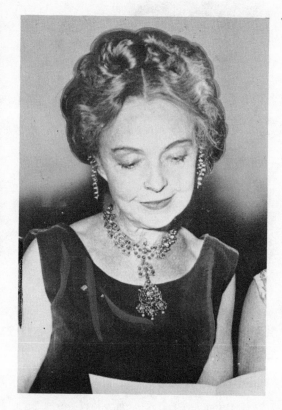

385

She appeared on the stage in Los Angeles with W. C. Fields, which led to many movie parts. She co-starred with Percy Kilbride in the *Ma and Pa Kettle* series.

1. *Marge Mainstreet.*
2. *Mary Tomlinson.*
3. *Marie Manheim.*

386

She is the distinguished "First Lady" of stage and screen. She won an Academy Award for her role in *Airport* and *The Sin of Madelon Claudet.*

1. *Helen H. Brown*
2. *Elizabeth Szatkowski.*
3. *Helen McHugh.*

387

A favorite of silent film devotees, she and her sister Dorothy were much-admired stars of the silent movies. She is also an accomplished stage actress.

1. *Lillian Gusher.*   2. *Lillian Garwood.*
3. *Lillian de Guiche.*

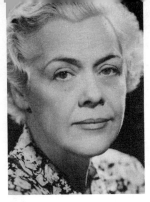

388

She was an American character actress who most often appeared in "ladylike" roles in early Hollywood films.

1. *Jeanette Beahman.*
2. *Janet B. Meysenburg.*
3. *Jan Beekman.*

389

If you have ever seen a movie, you must have seen this fine, angular British character actress. She has been in Hollywood for many years.

1. *Rachel Griffin.*   2. *Ethel Wood.*
3. *Gretchen Lehigh.*

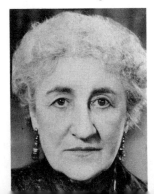

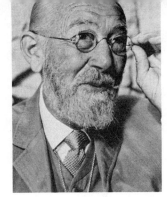

390

This suave Hungarian actor began in Hollywood as a romantic figure, then as a smooth villain, finally as a kind old man. He won an Oscar for *Watch on the Rhine.*

1. *Pal Lukacs.*   2. *Card Walker.*
3. *Paul A. Levi.*

391

This slightly built Canadian character actor of stage and screen is one of the nation's greatest actors. He is married to actress Jessica Tandy.

1. *Ron Cayo.*   2. *John Matlaga.*
3. *Hume Blake.*

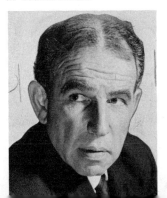

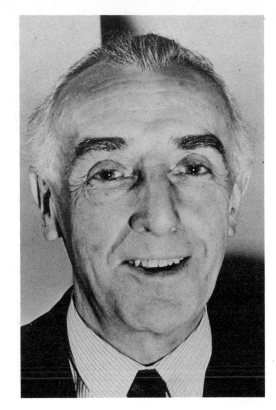

392

This fine American actor is best known for his stage role as Cyrano de Bergerac. He appeared in many Hollywood films, and was known as "The Grand Old Man of the Theatre."

1. *Walter H. Dougherty.*   2. *Paul Gerken.*
3. *Ara Parseghian.*

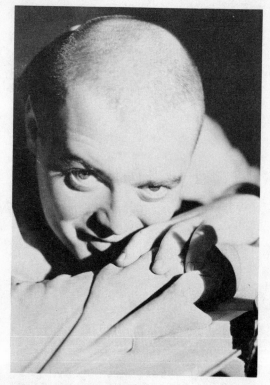

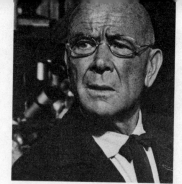

394

A fine American character actor who usually appeared in sympathetic roles; he was seen as colonels, fathers, town elders, etc.

1. *Dean Jeffries.*   2. *Robert Luzzi.*
3. *Ken Page.*

395

A great character actor on the American stage and screen. He is the father of director John Huston. Both won Academy Awards for their respective contributions to *The Treasure of the Sierra Madre.*

1. *Houston Walters.*   2. *W. Houghston.*
3. *Arnold Kopelson.*

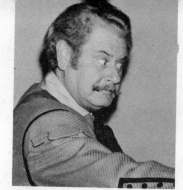

396

One of the most versatile of all Hollywood actors, this jovial, cheerful figure was a fixture in scores of films.

1. *Jon Davis.*   2. *Rufus Alan McKahan.*
3. *Lloyd Kaiser.*

397

This bald Polish character actor has entertained moviegoers since 1942.

1. *Mike Dann.*   2. *Jacob Keever.*
3. *Isser Kac.*

393

A Hungarian character actor whose "soft-boiled" eyes, timid manner, and unusual way of speaking brought him great roles with his friend Humphrey Bogart in *The Maltese Falcon* and other box office hits.

1. *Peter Lohrheim.*   2. *Lazlo Loewenstein.*
3. *Robert Luzzi.*

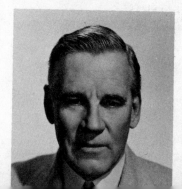

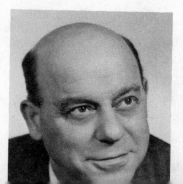

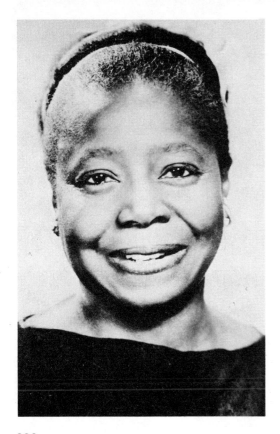

398

An actress with a most unusual high-pitched voice who appeared in *Gone With the Wind*. She started her career as a ballet dancer.

1. *Ada McQueen.*   2. *Thelma McQueen.*
3. *Queenie Brochner.*

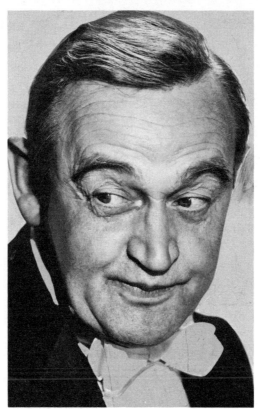

399

This fine character actor with an Irish brogue made a big hit with Bing Crosby in *Going My Way*, winning an Oscar for his performance.

1. *Lloyd Kaiser.*   2. *William Shields.*
3. *Mike Donovan.*

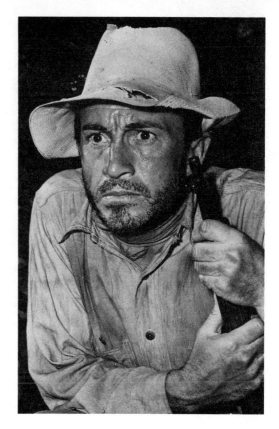

400

Here's an American actor who has played hundreds of roles as sheriffs, ranchers, doctors, etc., notably in *Giant* with James Dean.

1. *Norman Horowitz.*   2. *Paul F. Morrison.*
3. *Robert Henshaw.*

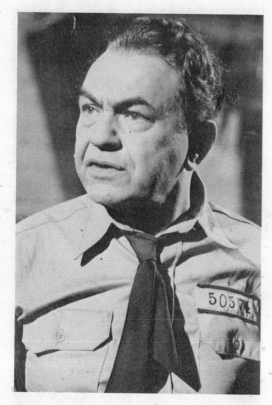

401

Here was one of the world's leading character actors. He began as an actor in the Yiddish theatre and became one of Hollywood's most popular actors.

1. *Emanuel Goldenberg.*   2. *Robert Henshaw.*
3. *Connel Murray.*

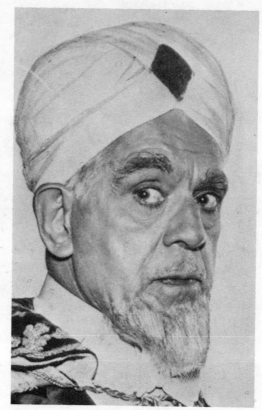

402

This British actor took the name of "Karloff" from ancestors of his mother. He enthralled and terrified millions of filmgoers.

1. *Vincent Donnely.*   2. *William Pratt.*
3. *William Urbanic.*

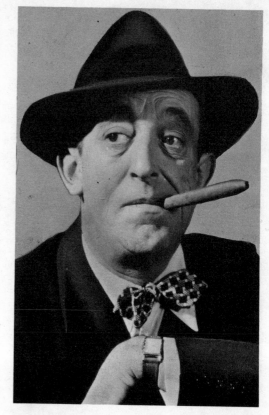

403

This "tough guy" American comic actor was a staple of the Warner Bros. repertory company in the thirties.

1. *Alfred McGonegal.*   2. *Bob Glickman.*
3. *Bobby Fleischer.*

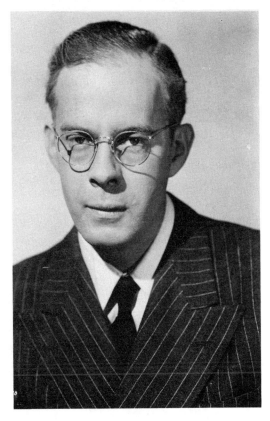

404

This great character actor is best known for his role on TV's hit series *M*A*S*H*. He has appeared in many Hollywood films.

1. *Harry Chomes.*   2. *Harry Bookhalter.*
3. *Harry Bratsburg.*

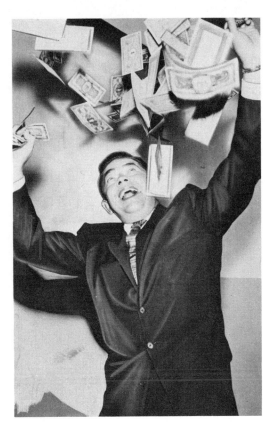

405

This talented actor began as a radio announcer and had a hit TV series, *The Millionaire*. He usually played tough-guy roles.

1. *Marvin Ziskind.*   2. *Leonard Marvin.*
3. *Marvin Mueller.*

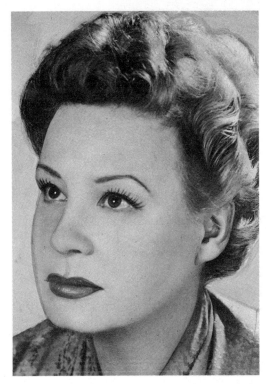

406

This Academy-Award-winning actress, for her role in *Come Back, Little Sheba*, is a distinguished American stage actress who usually plays middle-aged roles. She was a big hit on TV with *Hazel*.

1. *Thelma Ford.*   2. *Sherry Lansing.*
3. *Gladys Thurman.*

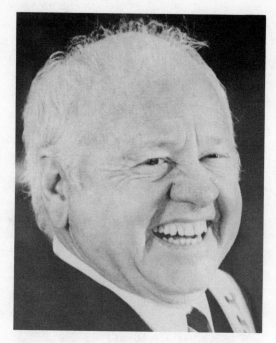

407

This dynamic, diminutive, aggressive, talented performer on stage, screen, and TV began in short comedies as "Mickey McGuire." He was outstanding in the film *Black Stallion*. He co-starred with Ann Miller in the stage hit *Sugar Babies*, and made many memorable films in Hollywood, especially the "Andy Hardy" series. He is a great entertainer.

1. *Myron S. Porter.*   2. *Joe Yule, Jr.*
3. *Jamie Dineen.*

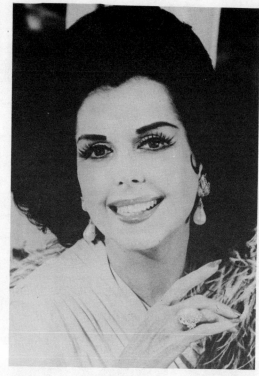

408

She's one of the loveliest and most talented of all stage, screen, and TV actresses. She's a fine dancer, known as "Queen of the Taps," and captivated millions as a comedienne and dancer in *Sugar Babies* on the stage.

1. *Anne Swedlow.*   2. *Annabelle Swanson.*
3. *Lucille Collier.*

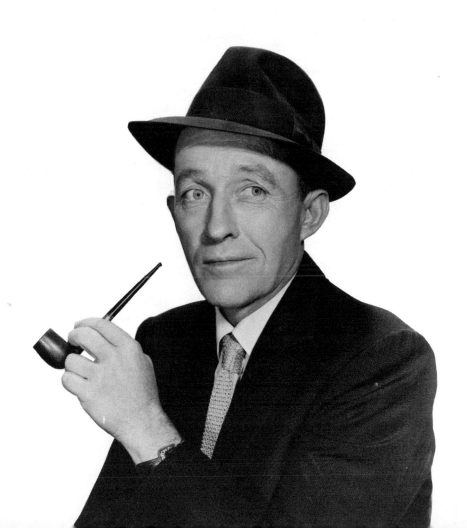

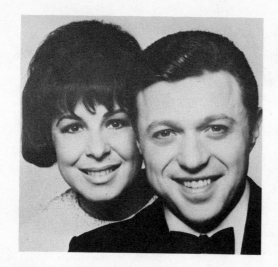

409

This multi-talented singer, actor, comedian is married to another talented singer-comedienne, Eydie Gorme. They are the darlings of stage, TV, and nightclubs.

1. *Sidney Leibowitz.*   2. *Steve Seymour.*
3. *Steve Yanovsky.*

410

This lovely singer is a fine comedienne. She and her husband Steve Lawrence are in great demand in fashionable clubs, on TV, and on stage.

1. *Edith Liebowitz.*   2. *Edyie Gorman.*
3. *Edith Gormezano.*

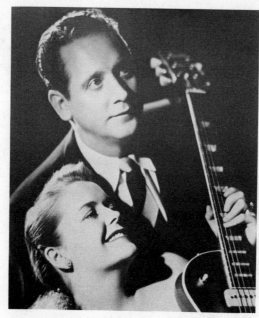

411

He was a great guitarist and recording favorite.

1. *Lester Zwiek.*   2. *Lester Polfus.*
3. *Lester Spitzer.*

412

She teamed up with Les Paul and they became a great team, in demand for radio, TV, and stage appearances. She married Les Paul.

1. *Colleen Summers.*   2. *Maria Carayas.*
3. *Mary Ann O'Dea.*

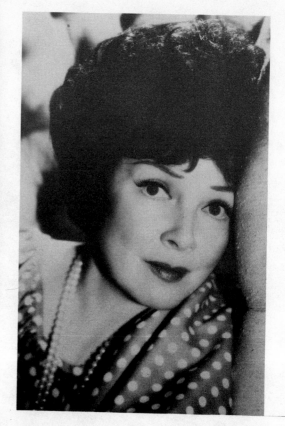

413

A great American singing star and musical-film favorite. She was one of "Andy Hardy's" dates in the popular movie series.

1. *Katie Valk.*   2. *Zelma Hedrick.*
3. *Kathryn Grey.*

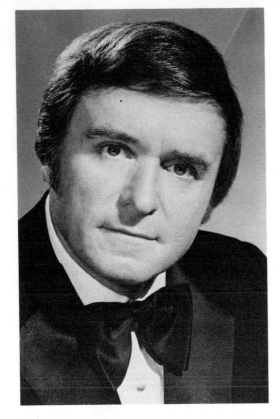

414

One of the nation's most popular talkmasters, he was a singer with Kay Kayser's orchestra.

1. *Michael Delaney Dowd, Jr.*
2. *Douglas Minhaelson.*
3. *John Murphy.*

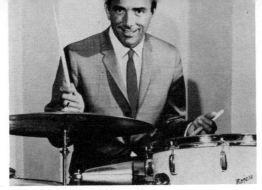

415

He is one of the world's best jazz drummers. He is married to Pearl Bailey, singer-actress of renown.

1. *Louis Bellassoni.*   2. *John Parrelli.*
3. *Roman Uzdejczyk.*

416

This gorgeous blonde was the leader of an all-girl orchestra. A vivacious entertainer, she was a great favorite in variety and musical specialties.

1. *Una Rae Hooten.*   2. *Odessa Cowan.*
3. *Bella Chaddis.*

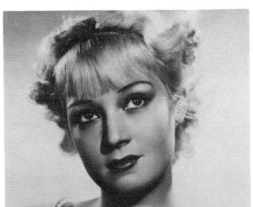

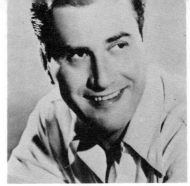

417

This great clarinetist is among the best-sounding big-name bandleaders ever. He once was married to Lana Turner, actress.

1. *Arthur Rosenfield.*
2. *Abraham Isaac Arshawsky.*   3. *Artie Baker.*

418

This handsome bandleader captivated thousands of listeners with his tantalizing music. He has done many films, also scoring them.

1. *Elliot L. Broza.*   2. *John Sousa.*
3. *John Connelly.*

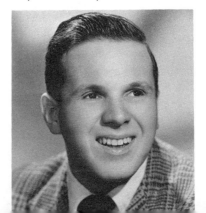

135

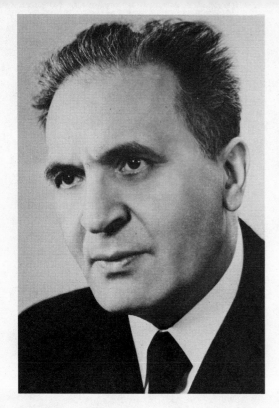

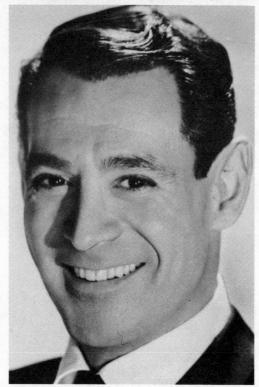

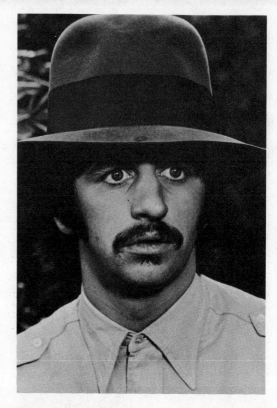

419

This brilliant maestro was a German conductor of major symphony orchestras throughout the world.

1. *Bruno Kaltenborn.*
2. *Bruno von Walterheim.*
3. *Bruno W. Schlesinger.*

420

This handsome bandleader was a favorite of millions who admired his special brand of music.

1. *Antonio Rybonnio.*
2. *Anthony Monello.*
3. *Ray Antonini.*

421

This popular British star was one of the Beatles. He changed his name in 1961. His nickname was given him by his mother, because he liked to wear rings.

1. *Robert Starwell.*   2. *Richard Starkey.*
3. *Ralph Sharkey.*

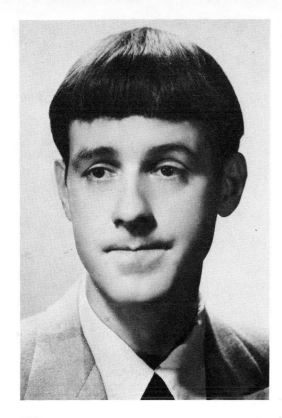

422

This musical comedian appeared with Kay Kyser's band, "The Kollege of Musical Knowledge," and was a popular figure among big-band audiences.

1. *John Gillick.* 2. *Peter Spengler.*
3. *Mervin Bogue.*

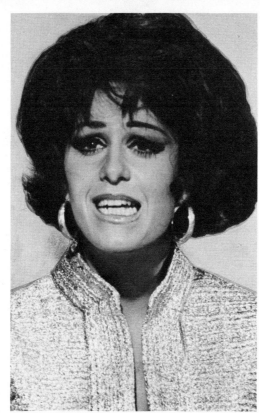

423

This bouncy, sultry American pop singer is a favorite of nightclub-goers everywhere. She appears frequently on TV and in films.

1. *Lanie Sherman.* 2. *Eleanor Stearns.*
3. *Lanie Levine.*

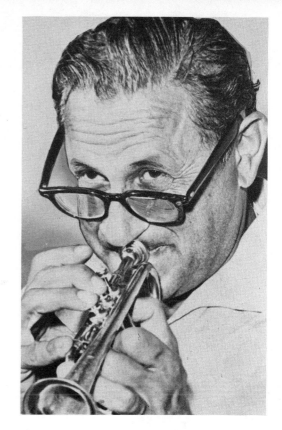

424

He was one of the famed jazzband trumpeters of the thirties and forties, and a favorite of music-lovers everywhere.

1. *Harry Finkleman.* 2. *Marty Ross.*
3. *Larry Gershman.*

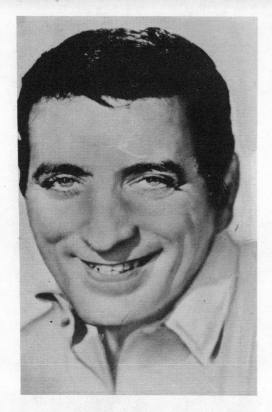

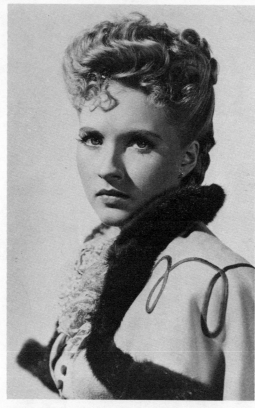

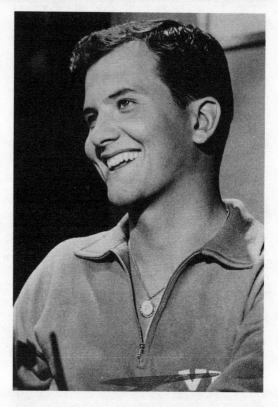

425

This American pop singer is one of the most versatile performers in the entertainment world. He is known by his trademark song, "I Left My Heart in San Francisco"—a gold record.

1. *Anthony Dominick Benedetto.*
2. *Angelo Picardi.*   3. *Tony D'Amelio.*

426

A leading American operatic singer and heroine of many films, she brought her beauty and talent to millions via the screen.

1. *Susan Frost.*   2. *Susan Larsen.*
3. *Susanna Finkel.*

427

This American pop singer is known for his "All-American-Boy" image and his white buckskin shoes. He is the father of singer-actress Debbie Boone.

1. *Daniel Boone.*   2. *Charles Eugene Boone.*
3. *Boone Patrick.*

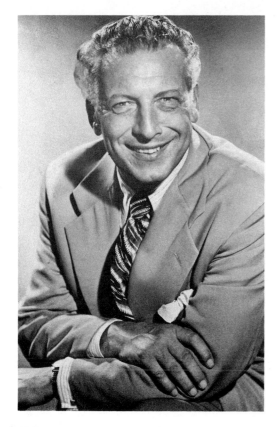

428

This handsome Italian opera singer's name became a household word with his stage appearance in *South Pacific* opposite Mary Martin.

1. *Fortunio Pinza.*   2. *Roman Matlaga.*
3. *Alan Silverbach.*

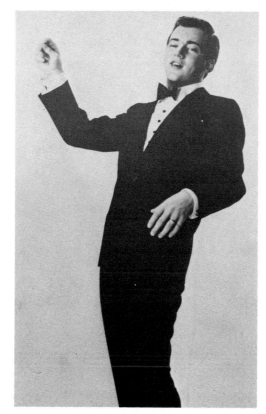

429

He was a dynamic singer who made several Hollywood films, notably *Pressure Point*. He was married to actress Sandra Dee.

1. *Jim Hergen.*   2. *Walden Robert Cassotto.*
3. *Bob Morin.*

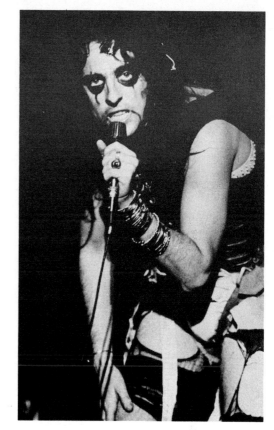

430

This American pop singer became famous in the mid-seventies for his sadistic stage act.

1. *Vince Furnier.*   2. *Vincent Musto.*
3. *Robert J. Scardina.*

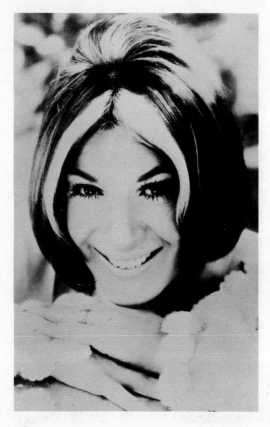

431

A popular singer whose unusual delivery has made her an international favorite. She appears in fashionable clubs and on TV.

1. *Vickie Carbarn.*   2. *Beth Waldorf.*
3. *Florencia C.M. Casillas.*

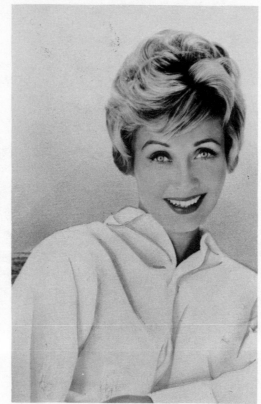

432

She is a diminutive American singing and dancing leading lady who was a child performer before becoming a Hollywood star.

1. *Suzanne Burce.*   2. *Jane Powers.*
3. *Oksana Glass.*

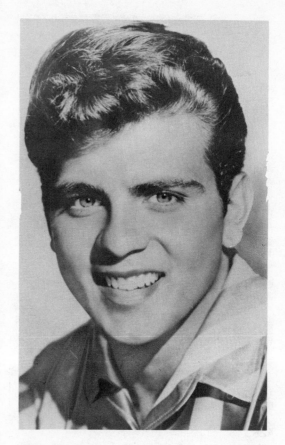

433

He is a fine American pop singer who had millions of followers in his heyday.

1. *Russ Fabian.*   2. *Joe Tirinato.*
3. *Fabian Forte.*

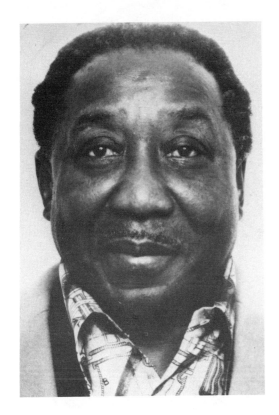

434

He's a fine American blues singer who has a big following among music lovers all over the world.

1. *McKinley Morganfield.*
2. *LeRoy Brown.*
3. *Joseph Fitzgerald.*

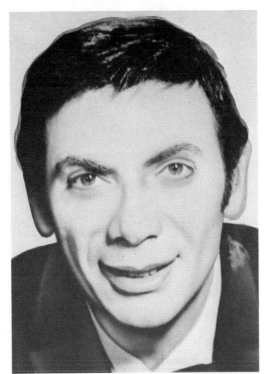

435

A remarkable singer and actor. He was one of The Ames Brothers and also made it big as a single, appearing in musical plays and on TV, where he played an Indian, "Mingo," in *Daniel Boone.*

1. *Edward Yorick*   2. *Morrie Roizman*
3. *Mike Moore*

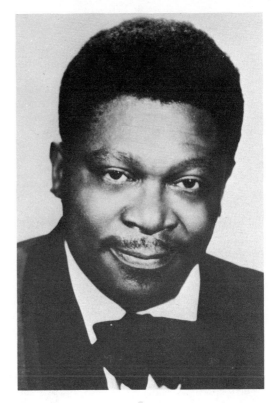

436

A famous American blues singer who started in show business as "Riley King, the Blues Boy from Beale Street." He retained the initials "B.B."

1. *Hamilton King.*   2. *King Fisch.*
3. *Riley B. King.*

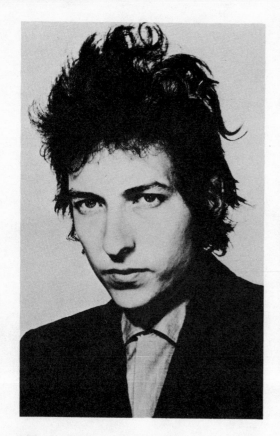

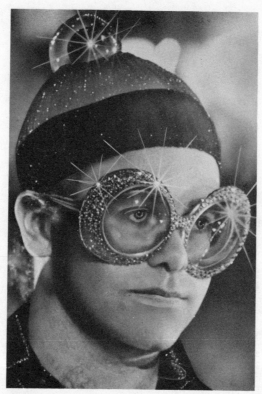

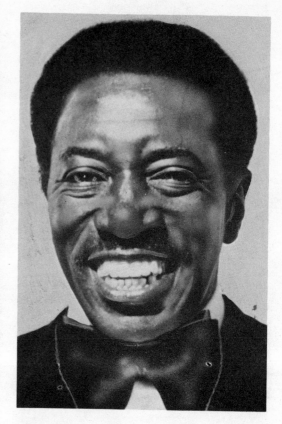

437

A great American pop singer, poet, and composer who officially changed his name in honor of Dylan Thomas, the Welsh poet.

1. *Bob Sheinfeld.* 2. *Robert Zimmerman.*
3. *Ed Briehn.*

438

A great pop singer who often wears bizarre clothes when performing before his millions of fans. He has innumerable platinum- and gold-record hits. He comes from Britain.

1. *Harold Banks.* 2. *Martin Oxer.*
3. *Reginald Dwight.*

439

A great singer known for his trademark of singing, "Oh, yeah!" He is considered to be among the best of American pop singers.

1. *William Josephs.* 2. *Joseph Matthews.*
3. *Joseph Goreed.*

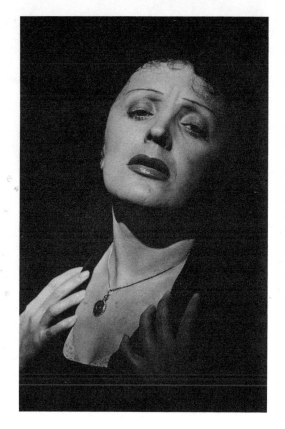

440

A great French songstress who became a legend among GIs during World War II. She changed her name to the French slang for "sparrow."

1. *Nanci Bonhomme.*   2. *Edith Gassion.*
3. *Hilda Speciale.*

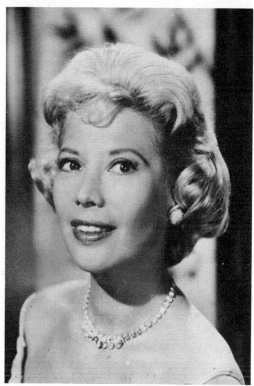

441

Beginning as a singer, she captivated American TV audiences with her own brand of humor and singing. She is an accomplished tennis player and hosted her own women's talk show on TV.

1. *Frances Rose Shore.*   2. *Dinah Saperstein.*
3. *Wendy Goldberg.*

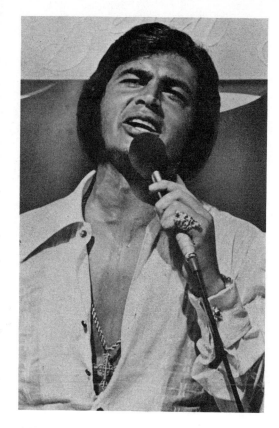

442

A great British pop singer who, like his counterpart, Tom Jones, is the darling of thousands of nightclub devotees.

1. *John Doscher.*   2. *Arnold Dorsey.*
3. *Frank Waldorf.*

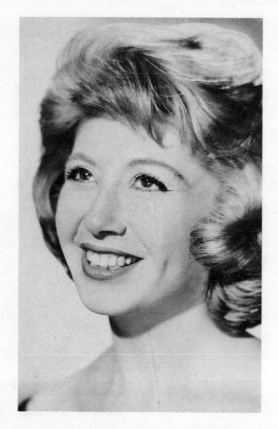

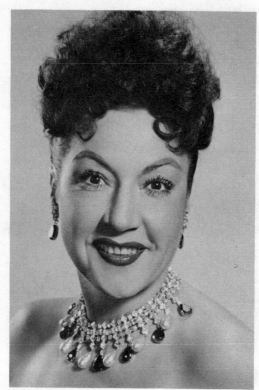

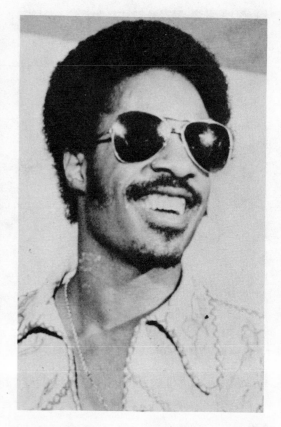

443

This great American opera singer began as a child prodigy and made motion pictures when she was a youngster. She now produces operas.

1. *Belle Silverman.*   2. *Beverly Silton.*
3. *Beverly Hilton.*

444

A great American musical comedy star whose voice is vibrant and brassy. She has an incomparable way of belting across a melody which has become her trademark.

1. *Etta Herman.*   2. *Ethel Zimmermann.*
3. *Ella Mermaid.*

445

One of America's greatest song stylists who attracts thousands of followers wherever he appears. His records sell in the millions.

1. *Stephen Judkins.*   2. *Joel Zaremby.*
3. *Stephen Wanderlust.*

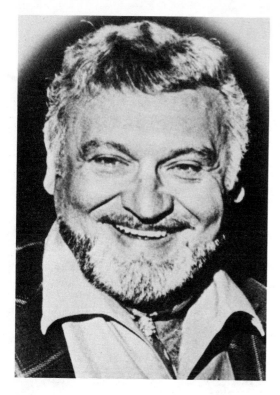

446

When this popular American singer started in show business, he changed his name to Laine when he discovered there was a singer named Frances Lane, so he added an "i" to make it different.

1. *Frank Lo Vecchio.*   2. *Lester Smith.*
3. *Robert DiPietro.*

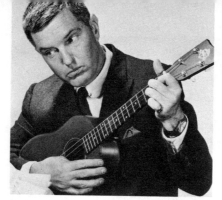

447

This handsome, talented singer entertained millions with his wife, Mary Healy, as a team during the fifties and sixties.

1. *Peter Potter.*   2. *Joseph Conrad Lind, Jr.*
3. *Tom Ettinger.*

448

This talented British cabaret songstress appeared in several films and starred on Broadway in *Oliver.*

1. *Lillian Klot.*   2. *Georgeann Taupe.*
3. *Joni Bass Brown.*

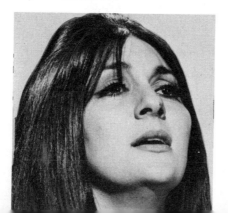

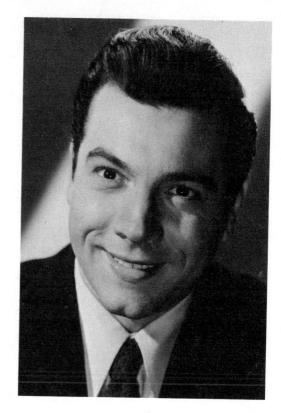

449

This American opera singer was popular in MGM musicals and made many successful movies in Hollywood. He even played the role of Enrico Caruso.

1. *Tony Balducci.*   2. *Alfredo Cocozza.*
3. *Bob LaRose.*

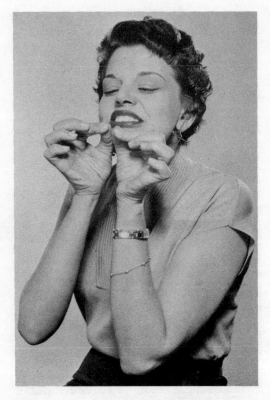

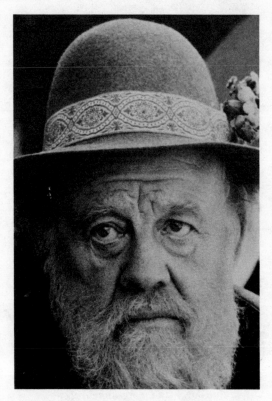

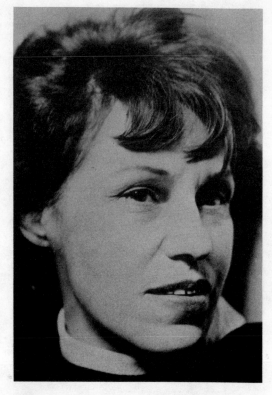

450

A fine American singer-comedienne with much stage experience. She starred in a fine TV series, *The Mothers-in-Law*.

1. *Cathy Roundtree*.
2. *Catherine Balotta*.
3. *Kathryn Mundane*.

451

A great character actor who began as a ballad singer and professional football player. He won an Oscar for his performance in *The Big Country*.

1. *Burl Icle Ivanhoe*.   2. *Terry Semel*.
3. *Ronald Sledge*.

452

This fine Austrian singer and actress married composer Kurt Weill and starred in his operas. She also appeared in *From Russia With Love*, a James Bond movie.

1. *Lotta Worque*.   2. *Caroline Blamauer*.
3. *Carmen Goinne*.

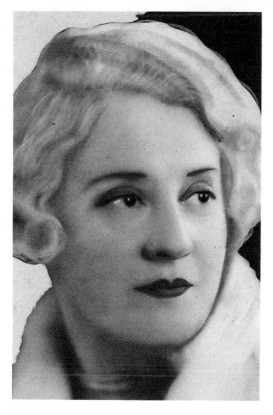

453

This lovely blond entertainer was a much-adored American vaudeville singer.

1. *Dora Goldberg.*
2. *Barbara Faison.*
3. *Marge Roedick-Barrack.*

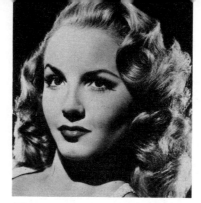

454

A beautiful and talented singer who contributed her talents to films and TV. She had a TV series, *The Smith Family*, in the early seventies.

1. *Joan Parks.*   2. *Martha Lafferty.*
3. *Jeanette Blohr.*

455

She's a fine musical comedy star who has appeared on the stage, screen, and TV with great success.

1. *Martha Washington-Lee.*
2. *Marsha Reichert.*   3. *Martha Wiederrecht.*

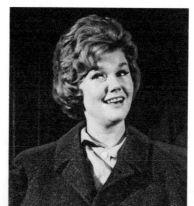

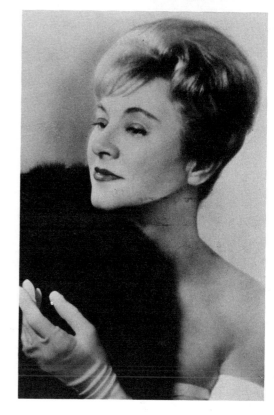

456

This beautiful, statuesque singer and pianist was the delight of cafe-goers and was a fixture on early radio programs. She was incomparable.

1. *Hildegarde Sell.*   2. *Hilda Klatdky.*
3. *Helen Grant.*

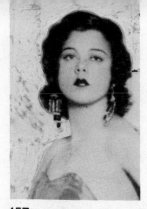

457

One of the world's greatest blues singers, who was swept to stardom during the thirties as the result of her sultry singing.

1. *Gertrude Gordon.*   2. *Leslie Evans.*
3. *Elizabeth Holzman.*

458

She was a great blues singer and had tremendous influence on those who followed her unique style of singing.

1. *Dinah Meitte.*   2. *Ruth Jones.*
3. *Donna Harris.*

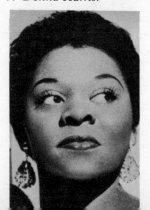

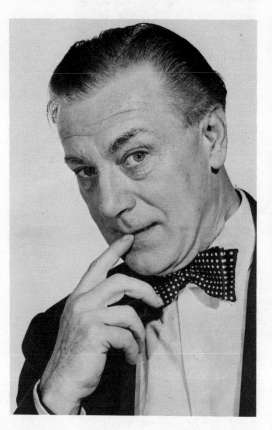

459

Here is a handsome British singer who made it big in American musical comedies. He is known for his great role in *The Vagabond King*.

1. *Dennis Pratt.*   2. *Jon Kay.*
3. *Jack Thayer.*

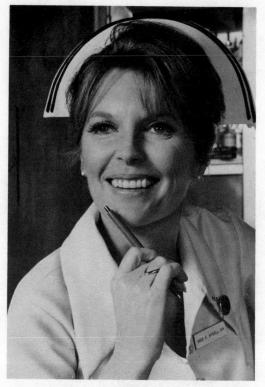

460

She is a popular singer who made millions happy by her role of "Dixie McCall" in the TV series *Emergency.* She has made many successful recordings.

1. *Julie Blankstein.*   2. *Julia Levine.*
3. *Julie Peck.*

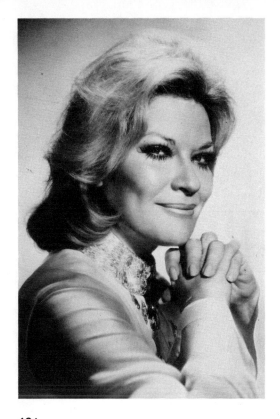

461

A grand American songstress, best remembered for her vocalizing of such hits as "In Old Cape Cod" and "How Much Is That Doggie in the Window?" She also appeared in films.

1. *Hallie Bieber.*   2. *Clara Ann Fowler.*
3. *Patricia Welles.*

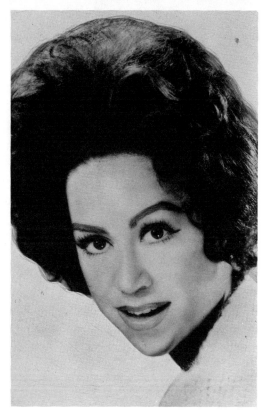

462

This beautiful American operatic soprano achieved international acclaim when she played the title role in *Melba* in the fifties.

1. *Patrice Munsil.*   2. *Patricia Mandell.*
3. *Patti Munseltry.*

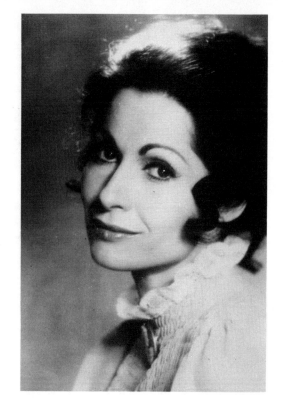

463

This beautiful American dancer and singer is well known for her commercials on TV as well as her frequent guest appearances on TV specials. She starred in the original *West Side Story*.

1. *Lorin Carlton.*   2. *Carol Laraia.*
3. *Carole Lorenzo.*

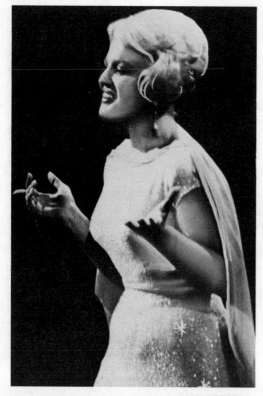

464

She is one of America's greatest song stylists. She appears in concerts and made an exciting appearance as the leading lady in *Pete Kelly's Blues* in Hollywood.

1. *Norma Egstrom.*   2. *Gertrude Morris.*
3. *Rebecca Weston.*

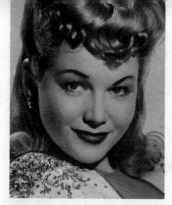

465

This vivacious singer was a leading lady in musical films of the forties.

1. *Mary Jane Frahse.*   2. *Janet Frazer.*
3. *Constantine Kazanas.*

466

This talented songstress made an important contribution to the American pop singing craze during the late sixties.

1. *Lisa Albrecht.*   2. *Carol Despres.*
3. *Joan Babbo.*

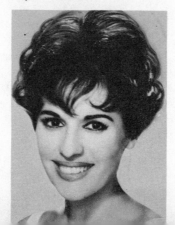

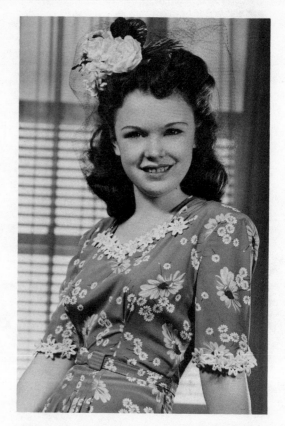

467

This lovely singer was a former child star who rivalled singer Deanna Durbin in the late thirties.

1. *Gloria J. Schoonover.*   2. *Gloria Batton.*
3. *Jean Gloram.*

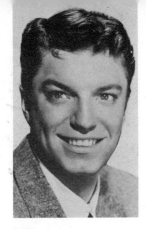

468

He's a stocky, boyish-type singer who thrilled millions during the fifties. He appeared in films and a TV series, *Whispering Smith*.

1. *Guy Parker.*   2. *Al Cernick.*
3. *John Fici.*

469

One of the Four Seasons, a popular singing group, who made it big on his own.

1. *Sid Berenson.*   2. *Frank Castellucciou.*
3. *Nat Buchman.*

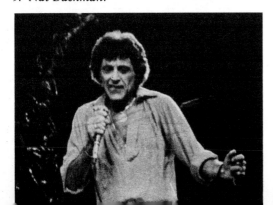

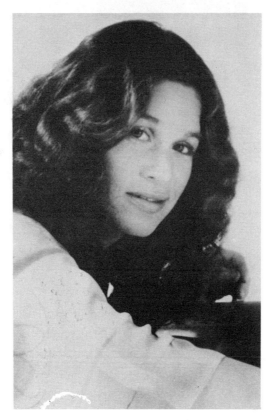

470

A great American pop singer and composer who plays to thousands at concerts and regularly makes gold and platinum records.

1. *Charlene King.*   2. *Carole Klein.*
3. *Charlotte Kingsman.*

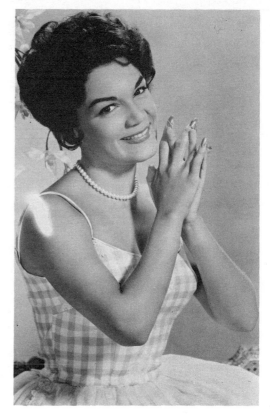

471

She's a great American pop singer who used her "reel" name for the first time on the *Arthur Godfrey's Talent Scouts* show in 1950.

1. *Connie Tutin.*   2. *Frances Constance.*
3. *Concetta Franconera.*

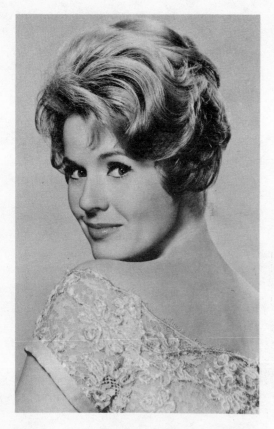

472

This beautiful singing actress is an American leading lady and stage actress. She is of Italian, English, Irish, and Mohawk blood.

1. *Andrea Chambers.* 2. *Joanne Dolinar.*
3. *Concetta Ingolia.*

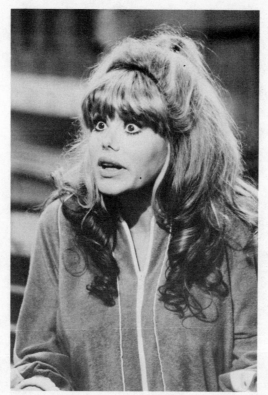

473

This "koochie-koochie," pert, petite singer-actress was once married to bandleader Xavier Cugat and appears on TV and in nightclubs, especially in Las Vegas.

1. *Rosita Charopilla.* 2. *Charlene Y Sabrina*
3. *Maria Rosario Pilar Molina Baeza.*

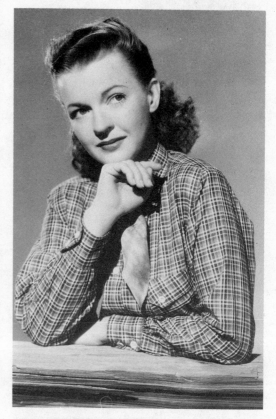

474

This beauteous lady rose from bandsinger to stardom in the forties. She married Roy Rogers in 1947.

1. *Frances Smith.* 2. *Frances Baker.*
3. *Monica Brethren.*

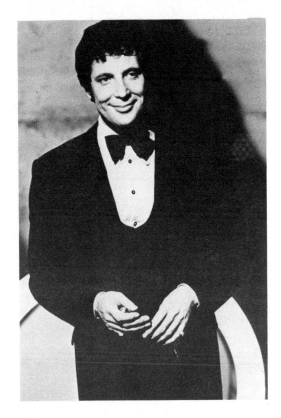

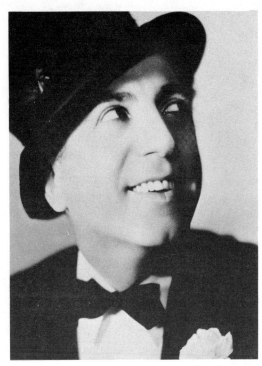

476

"Is everybody happy?" became a catch-phrase as uttered by this clarinet-playing orchestra leader. With his battered top hat and splendid showmanship he became an institution with American music lovers. His trademark was "Me and My Shadow."

1. *Theodore Friedman.*   2. *Theodore Factor.*
3. *Lewis Theodore.*

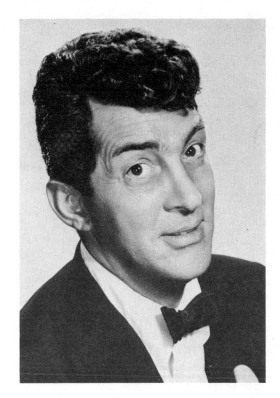

477

This handsome, self-spoofing American singer and leading man in films was teamed with comedian Jerry Lewis until 1956, then enjoyed spectacular success as a solo on TV, stage, and screen.

1. *Ray Goldman.*   2. *Dino Paul Crocetti.*
3. *Lee Barricino.*

475

This internationally famous pop singer was born in Pontypridd, Wales. He is the favorite of young and old alike, who revel in his singing and gyrations.

1. *Thomas J. Woodward.*   2. *Chuck Lanphear.*
3. *Marty Ross.*

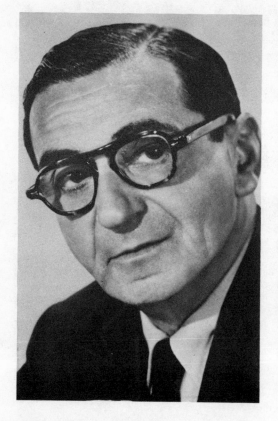

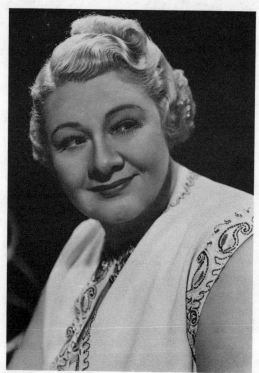

479.

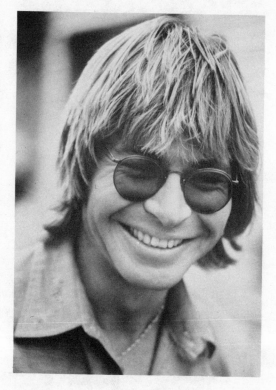

480.

478

One of the world's greatest writers of popular songs and probably the most prolific American composer and lyricist.

1. *Israel Baline.* 2. *Max Wilk.*
3. *Irving Shapiro.*

One of the greatest stage and vaudeville entertainers in American history. She was known as "The Last of the Red-Hot Mamas," and as a brash singer, she belted out songs like no one before her.

1. *Sophie Matlaga.* 2. *Sophia Kalish.*
3. *Sophia Abruza.*

He's a pop and folk singer and guitarist who has appeared in motion pictures with equally great success. He was a surprise hit in *Oh, God!* with George Burns.

1. *Henry J. Deutschendorff, Jr.*
2. *Clifford Rupprecht.*
3. *Johnny Moste.*

1. AL JOLSON, 2. *Asa Yoelson.*
2. JEAN HARLOW, 2. *Harlean Carpentier.*
3. LAUREN BACALL, 3. *Betty Joan Perske.*
4. LANA TURNER, 3. *Julia Turner.*
5. JOAN CRAWFORD, 2. *Lucille LeSueur.*
6. MARLENE DIETRICH, 3. *Maria Magdalena von Losch.*
7. CLARK GABLE, 2. *William C. Gable.*
8. WARREN BEATTY, 3. *Warren Beaty.*
9. JUDY GARLAND, 3. *Frances Gumm.*
10. JOHN BARRYMORE, 1. *John Blythe.*
11. GEORGE BURNS, 1. *Nathan Birnbaum.*
12. THE MARX BROTHERS, Groucho: 2. *Julius.* Harpo: 1. *Adolph.* Chico: 3. *Leonard.*
13. CARY GRANT, 1. *Archibald Leach.*
14. ROBERT REDFORD, 1. *Charles R. Redford, Jr.*
15. DANNY KAYE, 1. *David Daniel Kaminsky.*
16. EDDIE CANTOR, 2. *Edward Israel Iskowitz.*
17. BING CROSBY, 3. *Harry Lillis Crosby.*
18. BOB HOPE, 3. *Leslie Townes Hope.*
19. JACK BENNY, 1. *Benjamin Kubelsky.*
20. BARBRA STREISAND, 1. *Barbara Joan Streisand.*
21. GRETA GARBO, 1. *Greta Louisa Gustafson.*
22. LIBERACE, 1. *Wladziu Valentino Liberace.*
23. FRED ASTAIRE, 2. *Frederick Austerlitz.*
24. GINGER ROGERS, 1. *Virginia McMath.*
25. MARY PICKFORD, 2. *Gladys Smith.*
26. SOPHIA LOREN, 2. *Sophia Scicolini.*
27. RAQUEL WELCH, 1. *Raquel Tejada.*
28. VIRNA LISI, 3. *Virna Pieralisi.*

29. BO DEREK, 1. *Mary Cathleen Collins.*
30. MARILYN MONROE, 2. *Norma Jean Baker.*
31. RITA HAYWORTH, 2. *Margarita Carmen Cansino.*
32. ELKE SOMMER, 1. *Elke Schletz.*
33. CHERYL LADD, 2. *Cheryl Stoppelmoor.*
34. LINDA CHRISTIAN, 1. *Blanca Rosa Welter.*
35. SALLY RAND, 1. *Helen Gould Beck.*
36. CAROLE LANDIS, 1. *Frances Ridste.*
37. ANGIE DICKINSON, 1. *Angeline Brown.*
38. TWIGGY, 1. *Leslie Hornby.*
39. ANN SHERIDAN, 2. *Clara Lou Sheridan.*
40. RITA MORENO, 2. *Rosita Dolores Alverio.*
41. CAPUCINE, 1. *Germaine Lefebvre.*
42. LESLIE BROOKS, 3. *Leslie Gettman*
43. ZSA ZSA GABOR, 3. *Sari Gabor.*
44. DENISE DARCEL, 2. *Denise Billecard.*
45. CHER, 3. *Cherilyn LaPiere.*
46. JULIE NEWMAR, 1. *Julia Newmeyer.*
47. LILI ST. CYR, 1. *Marie Van Schaak.*
48. TERRY MOORE, 2. *Helen Koford.*
49. JOEY HEATHERTON, 3. *Davenie Johanna Heatherton.*
50. MORGAN FAIRCHILD, 2. *Patsy McClenny.*
51. DIANA DORS, *Diana Fluck.*
52. MAMIE VAN DOREN, 1. *Joan Lucille Olander.*
53. MAY BRITT, 1. *Maybritt Wilkens.*
54. KIM NOVAK, 3. *Marilyn Novak.*
55. CORINNE CALVET, 2. *Corinne Dibos.*
56. JAYNE MANSFIELD, 1. *Vera Jane Palmer.*
57. MARIE WILSON, 3. *Katherine Elizabeth White.*

58. SUZANNE SOMERS, 2. *Suzanne Mahoney.*
59. JAMES ARNESS, 2. *James Aurness.*
60. ROY ROGERS, 2. *Leonard Slye.*
61. JAMES GARNER, 1. *James Baumgarner.*
62. STEVE FORREST, 3. *William Andrews.*
63. GUY MADISON, 1. *Robert Moseley.*
64. VAN JOHNSON, 1. *Charles Van Johnson.*
65. BILL WILLIAMS, 3. *William Katt.*
66. GEORGE MONTGOMERY, 2. *George M. Letz.*
67. GENE NELSON, 3. *Eugene Berg.*
68. DENNIS O'KEEFE, 1. *Edward "Bud" Flanagan.*
69. GILBERT ROLAND, 3. *Luis Antonio de Alonso.*
70. CLINT WALKER, 1. *Norman E. Walker.*
71. MICHAEL LANDON, 1. *Michael Orowitz.*
72. GREGORY PECK, 3. *Eldred G. Peck.*
73. RAY MILLAND, 2. *Reginald Truscott-Jones.*
74. JOHN WAYNE, 1. *Marion M. Morrison.*
75. BUCK JONES, 2. *Charles Jones.*
76. ROD CAMERON, 1. *Nathan Cox.*
77. RANDOLPH SCOTT, 2. *George Randolph Crane.*
78. MICHAEL CAINE, 1. *Maurice Micklewhite.*
79. KARL MALDEN, 3. *Malden Sekulovich.*
80. TONY CURTIS, 1. *Bernard Schwartz.*
81. RICHARD BURTON, 1. *Richard Jenkins.*
82. WALTER MATTHAU, 1. *Walter Matuschanskayasky.*
83. WOODY ALLEN, 2. *Allen Stewart Konigsberg.*
84. CHARLES BRONSON, 1. *Charles Buchinski.*
85. JEFF CHANDLER, 1. *Ira Grossel.*
86. FREDRIC MARCH, 3. *Frederick McIntyre Bickel.*

87. ROBERT TAYLOR, 2. *Spangler Arlington Brugh.*
88. MIKE CONNORS, 3. *Kreker Ohanian.*
89. DON AMECHE, 3. *Dominic Felix Amici.*
90. ROBERT MONTGOMERY, 3. *Henry Montgomery, Jr.*
91. LOUIS JOURDAN, 2. *Louis Gendre.*
92. GARY COOPER, 3. *Frank J. Cooper.*
93. LARRY PARKS, 2. *Samuel Klausman.*
94. ROCK HUDSON, 3. *Roy Scherer.*
95. ROBERT BLAKE, 3. *Michael Gubitosi.*
96. MARTIN SHEEN, 2. *Ramon Estevez.*
97. EDDIE ALBERT, 2. *Eddie A. Heimberger.*
98. ALDO RAY, 1. *Aldo da Re.*
99. GEORGE BRENT, 2. *George B. Nolan.*
100. JON HALL, 3. *Charles Locher.*
101. PETER MARSHALL, 3. *Pierre LaCock.*
102. HUGH MARLOWE, 1. *Hugh Hipple.*
103. JOHN GAVIN, 2. *John Golenor.*
104. PETER GRAVES, 2. *Peter Aurness.*
105. LOUIS HAYWARD, 3. *Louis Woodward.*
106. ROBERT PRESTON, 1. *Robert P. Messervey.*
107. RORY CALHOUN, 1. *Francis Timothy Durgin.*
108. CLIVE BROOK, 1. *Clifford Brook.*
109. BRUCE CABOT, 1. *Etienne Pelissier de Bujac.*
110. ROBERT STACK, 1. *Robert Modini.*
111. OSKAR WERNER, 2. *Josef Bschliessmayer.*
112. DAVID WAYNE, 1. *Wayne McKeekan.*
113. SONNY TUFTS, 1. *Bowen Charleston Tufts III.*
114. TERRY-THOMAS, 1. *Thomas Terry Hoar-Stevens.*
115. GENE RAYMOND, 2. *Raymond Guion.*
116. JACK LORD, 1. *John Joseph Ryan.*
117. TELLY SAVALAS, 2. *Aristotle Savalas.*
118. BARRY NELSON, 1. *Robert Neilson.*
119. JACK PALANCE, 1. *Walter Palahnuik, Jr.*
120. RYAN O'NEAL, 2. *Patrick R. O'Neal.*
121. YVES MONTAND, 2. *Ivo Levi.*
122. JEFFREY LYNN, 2. *Ragnar Lind.*
123. JOHN LODER, 1. *John Lowe.*
124. MICHAEL WHALEN, 2. *Joseph Kenneth Shovlin.*
125. CLIFTON WEBB, 3. *Webb Parmalee Hollenbeck.*

126. GIG YOUNG, 2. *Byron Barr.*
127. JOHN DEREK, 1. *Derek Harris.*
128. TROY DONAHUE, 2. *Merle Johnson.*
129. OMAR SHARIF, 2. *Michel Shalhouz.*
130. JAMES DARREN, 3. *James Ercolani.*
131. JOHN FORSYTHE, 2. *John Freund.*
132. JOHN SAXON, 1. *Carmen Orrico.*
133. LESLIE HOWARD, 1. *Lazlo Steiner.*
134. TAB HUNTER, 1. *Arthur Gelien.*
135. VICTOR VARCONI, 1. *Mihaly Varkonyi.*
136. JOHN DALL, 3. *John Thompson.*
137. CHARLTON HESTON, 3. *Charlton Carter.*
138. ALEX CORD, 1. *Alexander Viespi.*
139. RICARDO CORTEZ, 1. *Jacob Kranz.*
140. JACKIE COOPER, 1. *John Bigelow.*
141. BUDDY EBSEN, 2. *Christian Rudolf Ebsen.*
142. CLAUDE DAUPHIN, 1. *Claude Franc-Nohain.*
143. STEWART GRANGER, 2. *James Stewart.*
144. TONY MARTIN, 1. *Alfred Morris.*
145. ROBERT ALDA, 3. *Alphonso d'Abruzzo.*
146. WILLIAM HOLDEN, 1. *William Beedle, Jr.*
147. KIRK DOUGLAS, 3. *Issur Danielovitch Demsky.*
148. ORSON BEAN, 2. *Dallas Burrows.*
149. VAN HEFLIN, 1. *Emmett Evan Heflin.*
150. WILLARD PARKER, 3. *Worster Van Eps.*
151. BRUCE BENNETT, 2. *Herman Brix.*
152. RICHARD ARLEN, 1. *Cornelius van Mattemore.*
153. ELLIOTT GOULD, 2. *Elliot Goldstein.*
154. JOHN GILBERT, 1. *John Pringle.*
155. JEAN GABIN, 1. *Alexis Moncourge.*
156. GLENN FORD, 1. *Gwyllyn Ford.*
157. PETER FINCH, 1. *William Ingle-Finch.*
158. ALAN YOUNG, 1. *Angus Young.*
159. YUL BRYNNER, 3. *Tadje Kahn, Jr.*
160. VINCE EDWARDS, 1. *Vincent E. Zoimo.*
161. BRUCE LEE, 1. *Li Jun Fan.*
162. JAMES CRAIG, 2. *James Meador.*
163. REX HARRISON, 3. *Reginald Carey Harrison.*
164. ANTON WALBROOK, 1. *Adolf Wohlbruck.*

165. HOWARD KEEL, 2. *Harold Keel.*
166. DOUGLAS FAIRBANKS, JR., 2. *Douglas Elton Ulman, Jr.*
167. GEORGE RAFT, 2. *George Ranft.*
168. SUSAN HAYWARD, 1. *Edythe Marriner.*
169. MALA POWERS, 1. *Mary Ellen Powers.*
170. PAULA PRENTISS, 3. *Paula Ragusa.*
171. ANNA MAY WONG, 2. *Wong Liu Tsong.*
172. POLLY BERGEN, 3. *Nellie Burgin.*
173. MARIE PREVOST, 1. *Marie Bickford Dunn.*
174. ELLA RAINES, 2. *Ella Raubes.*
175. VIRGINIA MAYO, 2. *Virginia Jones.*
176. JUDY HOLLIDAY, 1. *Judith Tuvim.*
177. CLAIRE TREVOR, 1. *Claire Wemlinger.*
178. MARGO, 2. *Maria Boldao y Castilla.*
179. SUSANNAH YORK, 1. *Susannah Yolande Fletcher.*
180. SIMONE SIGNORET, 3. *Simone-Henriette Kaminker.*
181. VERA HRUBA RALSTON, 1. *Vera Hruba.*
182. ANN SOTHERN, 3. *Harriette Lake.*
183. YVONNE De CARLO, 2. *Peggy Middleton.*
184. LILLI PALMER, 3. *Maria Lilli Peiser.*
185. GERTRUDE LAWRENCE, 2. *Alexandre Lawrence-Klasen.*
186. BETTY HUTTON, 3. *Betty Jane Thornburg.*
187. KAY KENDALL, 1. *Justine McCarthy.*
188. DORIS DAY, 1. *Doris Kappelhoff.*
189. DINA MERRILL, 2. *Nedenia Hutton Rumbough.*
190. KAREN BLACK, 2. *Karen Blanche Ziegler.*
191. KAREN MORLEY, 1. *Mildred Linton.*
192. STEFANIE POWERS, 2. *Stefania Federkiewcz.*
193. VERA MILES, 2. *Vera Ralston.*
194. IRENE PAPAS, 2. *Irene Lelekos.*
195. ANOUK AIMÉE, 3. *Françoise Sorya Dreyfus.*
196. POLA NEGRI, 3. *Appolonia Chalupek.*
197. JUNE ALLYSON, 2. *Ella Geisman.*
198. COLLEEN MOORE, 3. *Kathleen Morrison.*
199. BETSY PALMER, 1. *Patricia Brumbeck.*
200. DEBRA PAGET, 2. *Debralee Griffin.*
201. SHEREE NORTH, 1. *Dawn Bethel.*

202. JULIE ADAMS, 2. *Betty May Adams.*
203. ANDREA LEEDS, 2. *Antoinette Lees.*
204. CARA WILLIAMS, 3. *Bernice Kamiat.*
205. DEBORAH KERR, 1. *Deborah Kerr-Trimmer.*
206. HILLARY BROOKE, 2. *Beatrice Peterson.*
207. LILI DAMITA, 3. *Lilliane Carré.*
208. ILONA MASSEY, 3. *Ilona Hajmassy.*
209. SHIRLEY MacLAINE, 1. *Shirley M. Beaty.*
210. BINNIE BARNES, *Gitelle Enoyce Barnes.*
211. DIANA LYNN, 1. *Dolores Loehr.*
212. MITZI GREEN, 1. *Elizabeth Keno.*
213. KATHRYN GRANT, 1. *Katherine Grandstaff.*
214. ADELE MARA, 1. *Adelaide Delgado.*
215. COLLEEN GRAY, 1. *Doris Jensen.*
216. KIM HUNTER, 2. *Janet Cole.*
217. VIVIAN BLAINE, 1. *Vivienne Stapleton.*
218. LEE GRANT, 3. *Lyova Rosenthal.*
219. MICHELINE PRESLE, 1. *Micheline Chassagne.*
220. FRANCES DEE, 2. *Jean Dee.*
221. CLAIRE BLOOM, 3. *Claire Blume.*
222. JANE BRYAN, 2. *Jane O'Brien.*
223. EVA BARTOK, 2. *Eva Sjöke.*
224. NITA NALDI, 1. *Anita Donna Dooley.*
225. JEAN MUIR, 1. *Jean M. Fullerton.*
226. LYNN BARI, 3. *Marjorie Bitzer.*
227. WENDY BARRIE, 3. *Margaret Wendy Jenkins.*
228. MICHELLE PHILLIPS, 3. *Holly Michelle Gilliam.*
229. JEAN STAPLETON, 1. *Jeanne Murray.*
230. JAN STERLING, 2. *Jane S. Adriance.*
231. MARIE WINDSOR, 1. *Emily Marie Bertelson.*
232. DANA WYNTER, 2. *Dagmar Wynter.*
233. DONNA REED, 1. *Donna Mullenger.*
234. TALA SHIRE, 1. *Talia Rose Coppola.*
235. ROMY SCHNEIDER, 3. *Rosemarie Albach-Retty.*
236. LORETTA YOUNG, 2. *Gretchen Young.*
237. GALE STORM, 1. *Josephine Cottle.*
238. EVELYN BRENT, 3. *Mary Elizabeth Riggs.*
239. ELISABETH BERGNER, 1. *Elizabeth Ettel.*
240. BARBARA BRITTON, 2. *Barbara B. Czukor.*

241. DIANA WYNYARD, 1. *Dorothy Cox.*
242. ANITA LOUISE, 1. *Anita L. Fremault.*
243. SISSY SPACEK, 3. *Mary Elizabeth Spacek.*
244. BETSY BLAIR, 1. *Elizabeth Boger.*
245. AVA GARDNER, 1. *Lucy Johnson.*
246. LISABETH SCOTT, 2. *Emma Matzo.*
247. JANE SEYMOUR, 1. *Joyce Penelope Frankenburg.*
248. VERONICA LAKE, 2. *Constance Ockleman.*
249. MABEL NORMAND, 2. *Mabel Fortescue.*
250. BETTY FURNESS, 1. *Betty Choate.*
251. ARLENE FRANCIS, 2. *Arline Kazanjian.*
252. JOAN FONTAINE, 1. *Joan de Havilland.*
253. JEAN PETERS, 3. *Elizabeth J. Peters.*
254. MAUREEN O'HARA, 2. *Maureen Fitzsimmons.*
255. JUNE HAVER, 1. *June Stovenour.*
256. HARRIET HILLIARD, 3. *Peggy Lou Snyder.*
257. MARA CORDAY, 2. *Marilyn Watts.*
258. GLORIA GRAHAME, 1. *Gloria Hallward.*
259. VIRGINIA GILMORE, 1. *Sherman Poole.*
260. GAIL PATRICK, 1. *Margaret Fitzpatrick.*
261. HILDEGARDE NEFF, 3. *Hildegarde Knef.*
262. MAE MURRAY, 2. *Marie Adrienne Koenig.*
263. TALA BIRRELL, 1. *Natalie Bierle.*
264. MERLE OBERON, 1. *Estelle O. M. Thompson.*
265. MYRNA LOY, 1. *Myrna Williams.*
266. K. T. STEVENS, 2. *Gloria Wood.*
267. ONA MUNSON, 1. *Ona Wolcott.*
268. BLANCHE SWEET, 1. *Daphne Wayne.*
269. TUESDAY WELD, 1. *Susan Ker Weld.*
270. SHELLEY WINTERS, 1. *Shirley Shrift.*
271. DIANE KEATON, 2. *Diane Hall.*
272. PHYLLIS CALVERT, 2. *Phyllis Bickle.*
273. SANDRA DEE, 1. *Alexandra Zuck.*
274. JANE ALEXANDER, 1. *Jane Quigley.*
275. VALLI, 3. *Alida Maria Altenburger.*
276. VIRGINIA VALLI, 2. *Virginia McSweeney.*
277. LILA LEE, 1. *Augusta Apple.*
278. MARILYN MAXWELL, 3. *Marvel Maxwell.*
279. LINDA DARNELL, 3. *Manetta Eloisa Darnell.*

280. JANE WYMAN, 1. *Sarah Jane Fulks.*
281. AUDREY HEPBURN, 1. *Audrey Hepburn-Ruston.*
282. MONA FREEMAN, 2. *Monica Freeman.*
283. BRENDA MARSHALL, 2. *Ardis Ankerson.*
284. ANNA LEE, 1. *Joanna Winnifrith.*
285. JEAN HAGEN, 1. *Jean Verhagen.*
286. KIM DARBY, 2. *Zerby Denby.*
287. ANDREA KING, 3. *Georgetta Barry.*
288. DOLORES DEL RIO, 3. *Dolores Martinez Asunsolo.*
289. BRENDA JOYCE, 2. *Betty Leabo.*
290. GLORIA STUART, 1. *Gloria S. Finch.*
291. INA BALIN, 2. *Ina Rosenberg.*
292. ANN SHIRLEY, 1. *Dawn Paris.*
293. JEAN ARTHUR, 1. *Gladys Greene.*
294. PENNY SINGLETON, 3. *Dorothy McNulty.*
295. KATY JURADO, 2. *Maria Christina J. Garcia.*
296. LUPE VELEZ, 2. *Maria Guadaloupe Villalobos.*
297. JULIE ANDREWS, 1. *Julia Wells.*
298. JENNIFER JONES, 2. *Phyllis Isley.*
299. LOIS MAXWELL, 3. *Lois Hooker.*
300. JANIS PAIGE, 1. *Donna Mae Jaden.*
301. MICHELE MORGAN, 1. *Simone Roussel.*
302. CAROLE LOMBARD, 2. *Jane Alice Peters.*
303. BARBARA STANWYCK, 1. *Ruby Stevens.*
304. NATALIE WOOD, 1. *Natasha Gurdin.*
305. BARBARA BEL GEDDES, 2. *Barbara G. Lewis.*
306. ANNA NEAGLE, 3. *Marjorie Robertson.*
307. BESSIE LOVE, 3. *Juanita Horton.*
308. GILDA GRAY, 2. *Marianna Michalska.*
309. CYD CHARISSE, 3. *Tula Ellice Finklea.*
310. JILL ST. JOHN, 3. *Jill Oppenheim.*
311. PAULETTE GODDARD, 2. *Marion Levy.*
312. MILTON BERLE, 3. *Milton Berlinger.*
313. PHYLLIS DILLER, 1. *Ada Phyllis Driver.*
314. JACK OAKIE, 1. *Lewis D. Offield.*
315. SNUB POLLARD, 2. *Harold Fraser.*
316. LUPINO LANE, 2. *Henry George Lupino.*
317. BUDDY HACKETT, 1. *Leonard Hacker.*
318. BEN BLUE, 2. *Benjamin Bernstein.*

319. MARY WICKES, 1. *Mary Wickenhauser.*
320. JOEY BISHOP, 2. *Joseph Gottlieb.*
321. FRED ALLEN, 3. *John Florence Sullivan.*
322. BEN TURPIN, 2. *Bernard Turpin.*
323. GENE WILDER, 1. *Gerald Silberman.*
324. PHIL SILVERS, 1. *Philip Silversmith.*
325. RED SKELTON, 3. *Richard Skelton.*
326. KEN MURRAY, 1. *Don Court.*
327. ZERO MOSTEL, 1. *Samuel Mostel.*
328. CANTINFLAS, 3. *Mario Moreno.*
329. JACK E. LEONARD, 3. *Leonard Lebitsky.*
330. TOM EWELL, 1. *S. Yewell Tompkins.*
331. ARTHUR LAKE, 1. *Arthur Silverlake.*
332. JERRY LEWIS, 1. *Joseph Levitch.*
333. GARRY MOORE, 3. *Thomas Morfit.*
334. CHARLEY WEAVER, 1. *Cliff Arquette.*
335. MARTHA RAYE, 2. *Margaret O'Reed.*
336. FATTY ARBUCKLE, 3. *Roscoe Conklin Arbuckle.*
337. BUSTER KEATON, 1. *Joseph Francis Keaton, Jr.*
338. JACK CARTER, 1. *Jack Chakrin.*
339. SOUPY SALES, 2. *Milton Hines.*
340. REDD FOXX, 1. *John Elroy Sanford.*
341. PINKY LEE, 1. *Pincus Leff.*
342. RODNEY DANGERFIELD, 1. *Jacob Cohen.*
343. RED BUTTONS, 2. *Aaron Chwatt.*
344. STAN LAUREL, 2. *Arthur Stanley Jefferson.*
345. GEORGE O'HANLON, 1. *George Rice.*
346. BILLY BEVAN, 3. *William B. Harris.*
347. DON ADAMS, 3. *Donald Yarmy.*
348. LOU COSTELLO, 2. *Louis Cristillo.*
349. MRS. NUSSBAUM, 2. *Minerva Pious.*
350. VERA VAGUE, 1. *Barbara Jo Allen.*
351. CASS DALEY, 1. *Catherine Dailey.*
352. ED WYNN, 1. *Isaiah Edwin Leopold.*
353. EVE ARDEN, 1. *Eunice Quedens.*
354. FANNY BRICE, 2. *Fanny Borach.*
355. BEATRICE ARTHUR, 1. *Bernice Frankel.*
356. ELAINE MAY, 3. *Elaine Berlin.*
357. JOAN RIVERS, 1. *Joan Molinsky.*
358. TOTIE FIELDS, 3. *Sophie Feldman.*

359. MEL BROOKS, 1. *Melvin Kaminsky.*
360. FIBBER McGEE & MOLLY, 1. *Frank McGonagle (Fibber McGee).*
361. MOLLY, 2. *Marion Driscoll (Molly).*
362. AMOS 'N ANDY, 1. *Freeman F. Gosden (Amos),* 2. *Charles Correll (Andy).*
363. SPANKY McFARLAND, 3. *George Emmett McFarland.*
364. NANCY WALKER, 1. *Anna Myrthle Swoyer.*
365. VICTOR BORGE, 2. *Borge Rosenbaum.*
366. MIKE NICHOLS, 3. *Michael Peschkowsky.*
367. DANNY THOMAS, 1. *Amos Jacobs.*
368. SYLVIA SIDNEY, 2. *Sophia Kosow.*
369. JOSEPH CALLEIA, 1. *Joseph Spurin-Calleja.*
370. HOWARD da SILVA, 1. *Harold Silverblatt.*
371. SIG ARNO, 1. *Siegfried Aron.*
372. JOHN QUALEN, 2. *John Oleson.*
373. JOHN HOUSEMAN, 3. *Jacques Haussmann.*
374. MARIE DRESSLER, 1. *Leila Von Koerber.*
375. ESTELLE WINWOOD, 2. *Estelle Goodwin.*
376. GERTRUDE BERG, 1. *Gertrude Edelstein.*
377. BEULAH BONDI, 1. *Beulah Bondy.*
378. LOUIS CALHERN, 2. *Carl Henry Vogt.*
379. MELVYN DOUGLAS, 1. *Melvyn Hesselberg.*
380. SESSUE HAYAKAWA, 3. *Kintaro Hayakawa.*
381. STEPIN FETCHIT, 3. *Lincoln Perry.*
382. ARTHUR TREACHER, 2. *Arthur T. Veary.*
383. JANE DARWELL, 1. *Patti Woodward.*
384. AMANDA BLAKE, 2. *Beverly Neill.*
385. MARJORIE MAIN, 2. *Mary Tomlinson.*
386. HELEN HAYES, 1. *Helen H. Brown.*
387. LILLIAN GISH, 3. *Lillian de Guiche.*
388. JANET BEECHER, 2. *Janet B. Meysenburg.*
389. ETHEL GRIFFIES, 2. *Ethel Wood.*
390. PAUL LUKAS, 1. *Pal Lukacs.*
391. HUME CRONYN, 3. *Hume Blake.*
392. WALTER HAMPDEN, 1. *Walter H. Dougherty.*
393. PETER LORRE, 2. *Lazlo Loewenstein.*
394. DEAN JAGGER, 1. *Dean Jeffries.*
395. WALTER HUSTON, 2. *W. Houghston.*
396. ALAN HALE, SR., 2. *Rufus Alan McKahan.*

397. KURT KATCH, 3. *Isser Kac.*
398. BUTTERFLY McQUEEN, 2. *Thelma McQueen.*
399. BARRY FITZGERALD, 2. *William Shields.*
400. PAUL FIX, 2. *Paul F. Morrison.*
401. EDWARD G. ROBINSON, 1. *Emanuel Goldenberg.*
402. BORIS KARLOFF, 2. *William Pratt.*
403. ALLEN JENKINS, 1. *Alfred McGonegal.*
404. HARRY MORGAN, 3. *Harry Bratsburg.*
405. MARVIN MILLER, 2. *Marvin Mueller.*
406. SHIRLEY BOOTH, 1. *Thelma Ford.*
407. MICKEY ROONEY, 2. *Joe Yule, Jr.*
408. ANN MILLER, 3. *Lucille Collier.*
409. STEVE LAWRENCE, 1. *Sidney Leibowitz.*
410. EYDIE GORME, 3. *Edith Gormezano.*
411. LES PAUL, 2. *Lester Polfus.*
412. MARY FORD, 1. *Colleen Summers.*
413. KATHRYN GRAYSON, 2. *Zelma Hedrick.*
414. MIKE DOUGLAS, 1. *Michael Delaney Dowd, Jr.*
415. LOUIS BELLSON, 1. *Louis Bellassoni.*
416. INA RAY HUTTON, 2. *Odessa Cowan.*
417. ARTIE SHAW, 2. *Abraham Isaac Arshawsky.*
418. ELLIOT LAWRENCE, 1. *Elliot L. Broza.*
419. BRUNO WALTER, 3. *Bruno W. Schlesinger.*
420. RAY ANTHONY, 3. *Ray Antonini.*
421. RINGO STARR, 2. *Richard Starkey.*
422. ISH KABIBBLE, 3. *Mervin Bogue.*
423. LANIE KAZAN, 3. *Lanie Levine.*
424. ZIGGY ELMAN, 1. *Harry Finkleman.*
425. TONY BENNETT, 1. *Anthony Dominick Benedetto.*
426. SUSANNA FOSTER, 2. *Suzan Larsen.*
427. PAT BOONE, 2. *Charles Eugene Boone.*
428. EZIO PINZA, 1. *Fortunio Pinza.*
429. BOBBY DARIN, 2. *Walden Robert Cassotto.*
430. ALICE COOPER, 1. *Vince Furnier.*
431. VIKKI CARR, 3. *Florencia C. M. Casillas.*
432. JANE POWELL, 1. *Suzanne Burce.*
433. FABIAN, 3. *Fabian Forte.*
434. MUDDY WATERS, 1. *McKinley Morganfield.*
435. ED AMES, 1. *Edward Yorick.*
436. B. B. KING, 3. *Riley B. King.*

437. BOB DYLAN, 2. *Robert Zimmerman.*
438. ELTON JOHN, 3. *Reginald Dwight.*
439. JOE WILLIAMS, 3. *Joseph Goreed.*
440. EDITH PIAF, 2. *Edith Gassion.*
441. DINAH SHORE, 1. *Frances Rose Shore.*
442. ENGLEBERT HUMPERDINCK, 2. *Arnold Dorsey.*
443. BEVERLY SILLS, 1. *Belle Silverman.*
444. ETHEL MERMAN, 2. *Ethel Zimmerman.*
445. STEVIE WONDER, 1. *Stephen Judkins.*
446. FRANKIE LAINE, 1. *Frank Lo Vecchio.*
447. PETER LIND HAYES, 1. *Joseph Conrad Lind, Jr.*
448. GEORGIA BROWN, 1. *Lillian Klot.*
449. MARIO LANZA, 2. *Alfredo Cocozza.*
450. KAYE BALLARD, 2. *Catherine Balotta.*
451. BURL IVES, 1. *Burl Icle Ivanhoe.*

452. LOTTE LENYA, 2. *Caroline Blamauer.*
453. NORA BAYES, 1. *Dora Goldberg.*
454. JANET BLAIR, 2. *Martha Lafferty.*
455. MARTHA WRIGHT, 3. *Martha Wiederrecht.*
456. HILDEGARDE, 1. *Hildegarde Sell.*
457. LIBBY HOLMAN, 3. *Elizabeth Holzman.*
458. DINAH WASHINGTON, 2. *Ruth Jones.*
459. DENNIS KING, 1. *Dennis Pratt.*
460. JULIE LONDON, 3. *Julie Peck.*
461. PATTI PAGE, 2. *Clara Ann Fowler.*
462. PATRICE MUNSEL, 1. *Patrice Munsil.*
463. CAROL LAWRENCE, 2. *Carol Laraia.*
464. PEGGY LEE, 1. *Norma Egstrom.*
465. JANE FRAZEE, 1. *Mary Jane Frahse.*
466. JONI JAMES, 3. *Joan Babbo.*

467. GLORIA JEAN, 1. *Gloria J. Schoonover.*
468. GUY MITCHELL, 2. *Al Cernick.*
469. FRANKIE VALLI, 2. *Frank Castelluccio.*
470. CAROLE KING, 2. *Carole Klein.*
471. CONNIE FRANCIS, 3. *Concetta Franco.*
472. CONNIE STEVENS, 3. *Concetta Ingolia.*
473. CHARO, 3. *Maria Rosario Pilar Molina B.*
474. DALE EVANS, 1. *Frances Smith.*
475. TOM JONES, 1. *Thomas J. Woodward.*
476. TED LEWIS, 2. *Theodore Friedman.*
477. DEAN MARTIN, 2. *Dino Paul Crocetti.*
478. IRVING BERLIN, 1. *Israel Baline.*
479. SOPHIE TUCKER, 2. *Sophia Kalish.*
480. JOHN DENVER, 1. *Henry J. Deutschendorff.*